Gabriel Gaté's
GOOD FOOD FAST

Gabriel Gaté's
GOOD FOOD FAST

ANNE O'DONOVAN

First published in 1991 by
Anne O'Donovan Pty Ltd
56 Claremont Street South Yarra
Victoria 3141 Australia

Copyright text © Gabriel Gaté, 1991
Copyright photographs & drawings
© Anne O'Donovan Pty Ltd, 1991
Reprinted 1991 (twice)
Reprinted 1992 (three times), 1993

Written with Angie Burns Gaté
Edited by Marcelle Kerley
Indexed by Pamela Handasyde
Designed by Leonie Stott
Illustrated by Jacqui Young
Food stylist Ann Creber with Gabriel Gaté
Photographer Mark Chew
Set in Bembo by Bookset Victoria
Printed by McPhersons Printing Group Victoria

Cataloguing-in-publication entry
Gaté, Gabriel, 1955– .
    Gabriel Gaté's good food fast.

    Includes index.
    ISBN 0 908476 49 3.

    1. Cookery (Natural foods). 2. Health.
    3. Quick and easy cookery.
    I. Anti-Cancer Council of Victoria
    II. Title. III. Title: Good food fast.

641.563

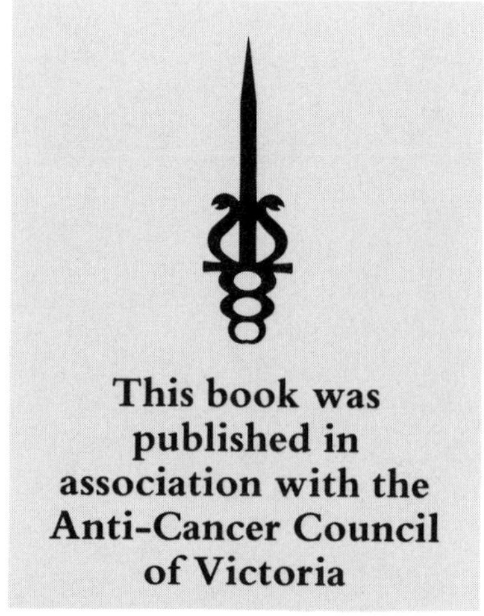

Cover photograph:
Healthy food in a hurry – quick-
cooking pasta tossed with vegetables
and garden-fresh herbs (page 61)

Foreword

'Good food fast' is not necessarily what your average consumer thinks of as fast food. Although the correlation between commercially available fast food and junk food is quite high, it doesn't have to apply to the food you cook yourself.

Most of us have a need to cook quickly from time to time and some of us have a need to cook quickly all the time. Gabriel Gaté, with his usual perception, has noticed this and is telling us how to go about it while still maintaining our standards.

Despite the fact that a lot of Australians eat poorly, there's very little excuse for this. Ours is a fertile country (at least, the part we choose to live in is fertile). It's probably also true that it needs a trip to another country for us to understand how uniquely fortunate we are in the way of natural produce. I always enjoy taking overseas visitors to the Prahran Market or the Victoria Market and watching them not only drool, but fall about in astonishment, at the variety and beauty of the food available.

Turning good materials, which are not necessarily expensive, into good food is a skill that anyone who can read can acquire. Given that we don't possess the miraculous facility that professional cooks have for preparation, we amateurs can nevertheless quite reasonably aspire to be good fast cooks.

Good Food Fast is the third book in the series produced by the fruitful collaboration between Anne O'Donovan, Gabriel Gaté and the Anti-Cancer Council of Victoria. The message has not changed. The Prudent Diet is still prudent and the diseases it helps to prevent are the same. However, this book has another creative attraction, and the easily prepared set of recipes ought to make it another bestseller.

Good Food Fast is a fun book and a simple one to read. But please don't overdo things; don't chop your finger off in cutting up the celery and, if you do, please don't add it to the stew.

Dr Nigel Gray
Director, Anti-Cancer Council of Victoria

Acknowledgements

I am happy to say that *Good Food Fast*, like my other books *Family Food* and *Smart Food*, has been a team effort. Working with friends, family and professionals in a range of fields has meant being able to produce a book that combines sensible nutritional advice with recipes that take into account how busy we all are today.

First of all I must acknowledge the ongoing advice, support and involvement of the Anti-Cancer Council of Victoria. The Director, Dr Nigel Gray, has been generous as always with his time and expertise. Many other people at the Council have offered professional assistance and encouragement. Of special note are Dr Robin Marks, Dr David Hill, Chris Keeler, Dorothy Reading, Marlene Rennie, Beverley Lovegrove, Pam Adams and Liz Tucker. Anti-Cancer Council staff have also assisted with testing the recipes.

Robin Hindson, Professor Kerin O'Dea, Dr David Topping and the Australian Nutrition Foundation have helped with additional information on nutrition. Ann Westmore has once again written an introduction that is informative and practical.

Special thanks to my publisher Anne O'Donovan, who has been committed to the project from the very beginning, and to her associates Margaret Barrett, Marcelle Kerley, Margaret Barca, Amanda Stephens and Pamela Handasyde; and to designer Leonie Stott, photographer Mark Chew, food stylist Ann Creber and her assistant Janet Lodge, and illustrator Jacqui Young.

As always, my biggest thanks go to my wife Angie Burns Gaté, who assisted with the enormous task of compiling and writing the book, but who is supportive in so many other ways. I must also thank Angie's mother Clare Burns, our sons Sebastian and Michael, and my brother Bernard Gaté.

Many of my friends and colleagues share my love of cooking and of good food and are more than willing in turn to share their knowledge and expertise – in particular Russell Morrison, Mary Jacobs, Sujatha Pannell, Terry Greguol (of Mario's greengrocer), Barbara Lord (from the Australian Conservation Foundation) and Rob Gell for information about being 'green in the kitchen'.

I must also acknowledge Elizabeth Chong, Theresa Janssen, Mary Larnach-Jones, Henrique Godinho from Casa Portuguesa, the staff at House in Carlton, the staff at Wedgwood, Bipen Sharma from Cafe Bombay and Heldi Bruce from Limoges for their help and generosity in providing cookware and accessories for the photographs in the book.

Gabriel Gaté

Contents

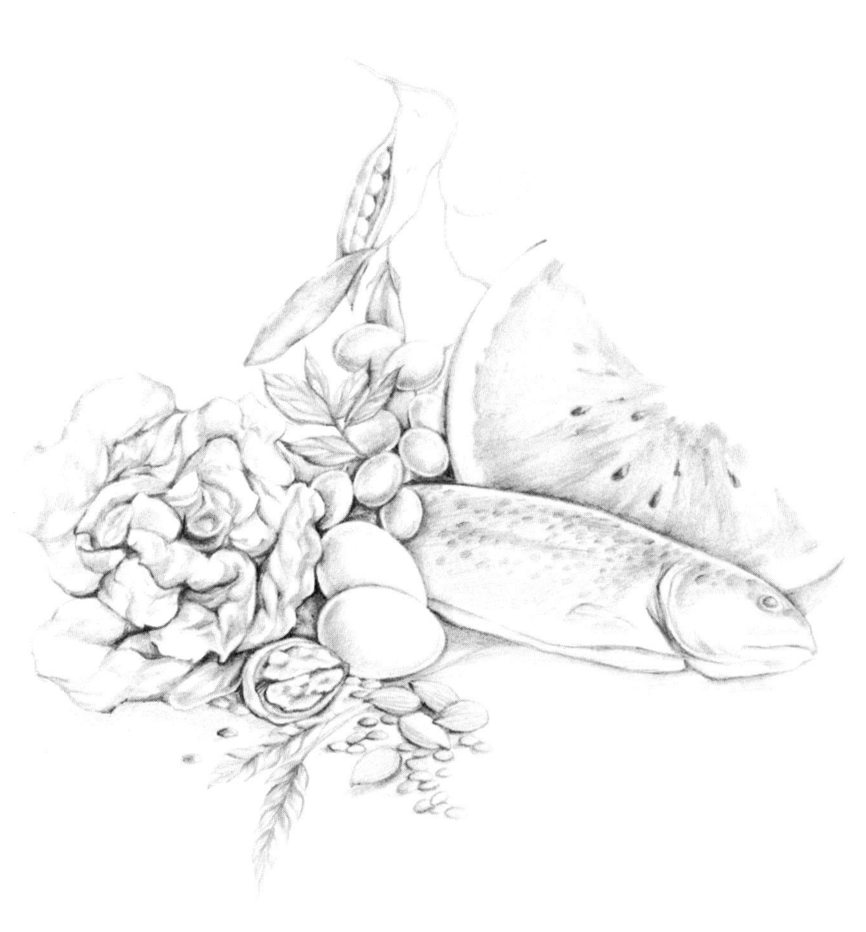

Variety – the Spice of Life

On your marks! Get set! It's time to start cooking good food fast.
Why fast? Because many people in Australia are juggling the
competing demands of work, family and leisure interests. They
have no wish to spend unnecessary time preparing or cooking food.
This is an unpalatable (to most cookbook authors) reality of
everyday life in Australia that deserves consideration.

It is a strength of Gabriel Gaté's approach to healthy eating that he
is realistic about the time, money and less tangible factors that
influence family eating in Australia.

One such 'less tangible' influence commonly occurs when we eat
out. Let us assume we are committed to healthy eating – less fat,
more fibre-containing foods, plenty of fresh fruits and vegetables,
less salt and sugar. How do we square our desire to eat nutritious
foods with the distinct possibility that what we will be served will
not fit the bill?

Gabriel Gaté's philosophy of life puts great emphasis on the
importance of sharing food and enjoying the company of friends,
family and colleagues. Such opportunities should be welcomed for
the pleasures they bring, not feared because of what they may do to
the waistline, hips or heart. The whole aim of eating healthily is not
to induce guilt or anxiety but to enhance our sense of well-being and
to heighten our enjoyment both in the short term and in the future.

If you are able to choose what you eat and drink when dining out,
by all means select judiciously in line with the Prudent Diet.
However, if the salad arrives swamped in dressing, the vegetables
are coated in a rich sauce, and the fish has been fried instead of
grilled, don't despair. What counts in terms of good health is the
type of food we eat most of the time. The occasional departure from
the norm will not create havoc with our weight or well-being. At
other times, when we have more control over the situation, we can
enjoy the crispest, freshest, leanest, most multigrained goodies
available.

Australian health authorities, including State cancer councils, the
National Heart Foundation, diabetes organisations and government
health departments, consider that we should apply the same sort of
common-sense approach when selecting the ingredients for meals.

There may be times, for instance, when our budgets cannot cope
with the cost of particular ingredients. Once again, be positive and
flexible. Look around for seasonal produce. It will be fresh, bursting
with flavour, full of vitamins and minerals and, importantly, it will
be kind to the pocket. Then find a recipe that suits the good-value-
for-money ingredients you have purchased and the time you have
available. This is part of the adventure of eating.

Liberated from preconceived ideas, we may end up selecting
something we have rarely or never tried, and this encourages the
variety and balance that form key elements of the Prudent Diet.

It is encouraging to see many Australians making dietary changes
in line with current advice from health authorities. These consumers
are eating less fat and salt, and drinking less alcohol. They are
leading the charge on butchers for leaner cuts of meat and are
dreaming up innovative ways of including some fruit and vegetables
in every meal.

At the same time, these consumers are in the forefront of those making greater use of seasonal and regional produce. In the warmest months, they stack their shopping baskets with the abundant and refreshing cantaloupes and watermelons, firm young bananas and sweet berry fruits. In the coolest months, they make good use of Australia's excellent supply of vitamin-rich oranges and mandarins and of hearty vegetables such as broccoli.

Building on the advice given in *Good Food Fast*'s predecessors, *Family Food* and *Smart Food*, Gabriel Gaté shows how anyone with an interest in food can quickly and economically produce healthy dishes full of flavour, texture and colour. There is no luck involved, even for beginner cooks.

All the recipes are based on thorough research and testing. They reflect the need for balance and variety. Our bodies need a mixture of foods from each of the five food groups: breads and cereals; vegetables and fruit; meat, fish, eggs, poultry or legumes; milk, cheese or yoghurt; and butter or margarine.

Federal health authorities have mapped out a food guide for good health. Each day you should aim to eat the following.

- Four servings of bread or cereals to provide food energy, dietary fibre (roughage), proteins, some vitamins and minerals. Choose from bread, ready-to-eat and cooked cereal, rice and pasta. Select wholegrain products for preference.
- Four servings of vegetables and fruit to provide vitamins and minerals and dietary fibre. Choose one serving that is dark green, yellow or orange (for example, broccoli, carrots, pumpkin, apricots, cantaloupe or mango), one from the citrus, tropical, tomato or berry fruit families, and two servings of any other vegetables or fruit.
- One serving of meat or meat alternatives to provide protein for muscles, iron for blood, and other minerals and vitamins. Choose from beef, veal, lamb, poultry, eggs, fish, dried peas and beans, lentils, nuts and peanut butter.
- 300 ml for adults, 600 ml for children and expectant or nursing mothers of milk and milk products to provide calcium for bones and teeth structure, some vitamins and protein. Choose from fluid, evaporated or powdered milk, yoghurt and cheeses or low-fat dairy products.
- One tablespoon only of butter, margarine or cooking oil to provide vitamin A and food energy. Cream can be substituted occasionally (one tablespoon of butter or margarine is equivalent to two tablespoons of cream).

About half of the kilojoules (energy) in a meal should be supplied by foods rich in complex carbohydrates. This is because they are more slowly digested and provide a more even energy release in the period between meals than do other foods. Breads and cereals rich in complex carbohydrates also contain vitamins, minerals and fibre that are essential for a balanced diet.

The fat content of meals should provide less than a third of the kilojoules. Fat is the most energy-dense type of food and if we consume more energy than we need, the extra will be stored as fat, leading to weight gain. Nutritionists recommend that the remaining kilojoules in the diet (about 15 per cent) should come from protein.

While there is evidence of encouraging nutritional changes among some groups in Australia, too many people continue to eat in a way

that is incompatible with good health. Lavish and constant
television food advertising targeted at children as well as adults
promotes excessive consumption of sweet, salty and fatty foods as a
key element in an exciting life-style. It is time to tackle this situation
as we work towards:

- cutting back on fats, sugar, salt and alcohol
- increasing our intake of complex carbohydrate and fibre-rich
  foods such as wholegrain breads and pasta, cereals, legumes,
  fruits and vegetables
- ensuring that we eat a wide variety of foods

The benefits to be expected include a substantial reduction in the
risk of heart disease, stroke, high blood pressure, anaemia, adult-
onset diabetes, diverticulitis, haemorrhoids, constipation and weight
disorders.

A well-balanced diet also has implications for reducing the risk of
developing certain types of cancer. Indeed nutrition is the new buzz
word in cancer prevention circles, with the release of authoritative
findings about the anti-cancer benefits of cutting fat consumption
and eating more fresh fruit and vegetables. There is strong evidence
that what we eat influences our risk of developing cancers of the
bowel, stomach, prostate, breast, endometrium and pancreas.
Among smokers, daily consumption of green and yellow vegetables
seems to have a protective effect by reducing the risk of developing
lung cancer and, in women, cervix cancer. International cancer
authorities estimate that of all cancer deaths in Australia each year,
about 35 per cent (that is, over 8000 deaths) are influenced in some
way by diet.

Looking beyond cancer to all deaths in the Australian population,
it is estimated that diet-related diseases account for up to 60 per cent
of the total in one way or another. These diseases are also linked to
other life-style factors such as smoking and inactivity, and it seems
that some people's genetic make-up multiplies the detrimental
impact of a poor diet, which in turn interacts with smoking and lack
of exercise.

The organic food movement in Australia reflects a widespread
concern that our food supply is at risk of losing some of its
freshness, flavour, and freedom from contamination. Eating a diet
with plenty of variety, while steering clear of excess, guards against
the major nutrition-related diseases in Australia. It also helps to
ensure that a deficiency or contaminant in a particular type of
produce will not lead to significant harm to the consumer.

As increasing numbers of people discover how enjoyable a
healthy diet can be, they are also acknowledging that there is no
need for food faddism and dietary extremes.

Together with Gabriel Gaté, I encourage all readers to enjoy the
experience of *Good Food Fast*'s quick-to-prepare, common-sense,
low-cost dishes.

Ann Westmore

The Prudent Diet

The recipes and technical advice in this book are based on the following recommendations.*

1   Make sure you eat a wide variety of foods

2   Control your weight: avoid obesity

3   Cut down on total fat intake

4   Eat more high-fibre and micronutrient-rich foods (fruits, vegetables, wholegrain cereal products). Make sure you include plenty of leafy green and yellow vegetables such as spinach and carrots, and members of the cabbage family such as brussels sprouts and broccoli

5   Eat moderate quantities only of salt-cured, smoked and nitrite-cured foods

6   Limit alcohol intake

*Because heart authorities advise a lowered salt intake in addition to the preceding recommendations, the recipes incorporate this dietary strategy.

NOTE: In recipes where cup measurements are indicated, a metric cup (250 ml or 8½ oz) should be used.

Good Food Fast

At the end of a busy day when I am a bit tired and the children are 'starving', I look at the clock and ask myself, 'How long will it take me to prepare a satisfying dinner?' More than ever the challenge for the busy home cook in the 1990s is to prepare good food fast. Good food needs to be varied, appetising, flavoursome and nutritious, and these qualities are quite compatible with fast cooking.

In this book you will find cooking tips, descriptions of quick techniques, and over 160 recipes that do not take long to prepare. If you have some experience in the kitchen, you will find that by using this book you'll be able to prepare most dishes in fewer than thirty minutes. And remember that every new dish will be faster to make the second and third time around. A confident cook is a fast cook. Novice cooks will greatly benefit from taking up the cookery course contained in chapter 2. It introduces easy, delicious dishes and simple cookery techniques and advises on shopping and choosing cookware. Towards the end of the book parents will find ideas to help their children become happy eaters and happy cooks, and there are a few recipes for the kids to try.

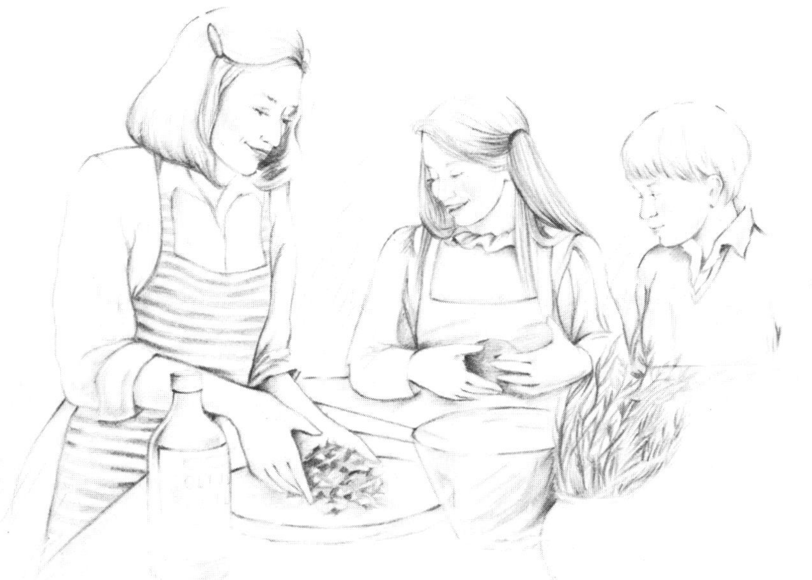

Cooking is an activity that should be carried out in a relaxed mood and, if feeling tense, I find it worthwhile spending a few minutes calmly putting my thoughts together. I might change into comfortable shoes, have a spell in the garden or lie down for a few minutes. Once relaxed, I cook more quickly and efficiently and derive greater pleasure from it.

Getting children to help is a great time-saver. Meal times are a time for talking, solving little problems and bringing the family together. As the children grow older and more skilful in the kitchen, we appreciate their help more and more, and no doubt they will be grateful for what they are now learning.

A fast kitchen

Always have canned tomatoes on hand. They can be a short cut to many delicious vegetable dishes, soups and sauces.

The prime asset of a kitchen is enough free bench space for preparing and serving food efficiently, and I consider one and a half metres of bench space to be a minimum to prepare food for a household of four people. But a spacious bench top does not necessarily mean a spacious kitchen. In fact, most cooks find a kitchen more comfortable to work in when the stove, fridge and sink are close to one another. Good lighting is another must in a kitchen, as is a generous-sized pantry that allows for the storage of a wide variety of easily and quickly prepared ingredients, such as pasta, rice, canned foods and potatoes. Dry foods, like flour, sugar and breadcrumbs, are more easily located when stored in clearly labelled containers.

To save time and energy, saucepans, oven dishes, trays and tins are best kept next to the stove and oven. Mixing bowls and small equipment can be stored under the work bench or hung alongside it. Of all cooking preparations, cutting and trimming take the longest time, so good-quality, sharp knives are a bonus to every cook. I like to keep my knives in a knife block on the work bench and keep them sharp by using a sharpening steel and by occasionally using a stone. (Professional knife sharpeners are listed in the telephone book.) A medium to large chopping board made of wood is my preferred cutting surface as it has a pleasant feel to it. I would spend more time in my kitchen if it were not for my food processor. It is a great timesaver in blending soups, puréeing vegetables and making sauces smooth, and it also cuts, shreds and chops vegetables, mixes cakes and performs many other tasks. I do find it quicker to use a knife when chopping a small quantity of parsley or an onion, as a knife is easier to wash than a food processor. It is advisable to use saucepans with well-fitting lids and to select the size appropriate to the quantity of food you are cooking. In a large wok you can enjoy preparing many one-pot dishes in no time at all, while a large steamer allows you to cook the lightest meal, including

Look for fruits canned in natural juices. They are an excellent pantry standby for healthy desserts in a hurry.

meats, vegetables and potatoes, with a minimum of effort. Remember that a hearty casserole takes less time to cook in a pressure cooker. Also, when you are using a traditional oven, preheat it for a few minutes to save on cooking time. Although microwave ovens can't cook everything, they do cook food rapidly, especially in small quantities, and they thaw food well. Many other small details, such as the position of the rubbish bin, can make your kitchen more efficient and a joy to work in. Make sure that children and partners know where to find things, especially teatowels and sponges!

Shopping for food

Our home cooking is the result of carefully selected ingredients quickly prepared to make a wholesome meal. An organised approach to shopping makes things work more conveniently. As with the cooking, it is always easier if the shopping is shared between household members. At our place, my wife Angie and I make lists of things we need and, to save time, we try to shop on the way back from work, leisure or other activities. Shopkeepers are aware that most home cooks have less time to spend in the kitchen than they did in the past and so try to simplify our tasks by offering a wider service. Butchers offer small, lean cuts of meat that require less time to cook and poulterers are happy to portion chicken in a dozen different ways to help save time. Fishmongers will clean, scale, fillet or cut your fish the way you want it, and this may save ten minutes in the preparation of a dish. I have found that we benefit greatly from fostering a friendly, open relationship with the people from whom we buy fresh food. We need them and they need us.

What to keep in the pantry and the refrigerator

As we all enjoy different foods, it would be inappropriate for me to suggest which foods to have on hand in your pantry, fridge or freezer. However, it may be useful to list the groups of foods that are convenient to have at the ready and that will help speed up the preparation of many dishes in this book. It is important to read labels carefully in order to understand the content of the food you buy and to select food low in added fat, salt and sugar.

IN THE PANTRY
- Pasta of various shapes (preferably wholemeal), rice (preferably brown), other cereals, such as barley, bourghul, couscous, polenta and, of course, breakfast cereals.

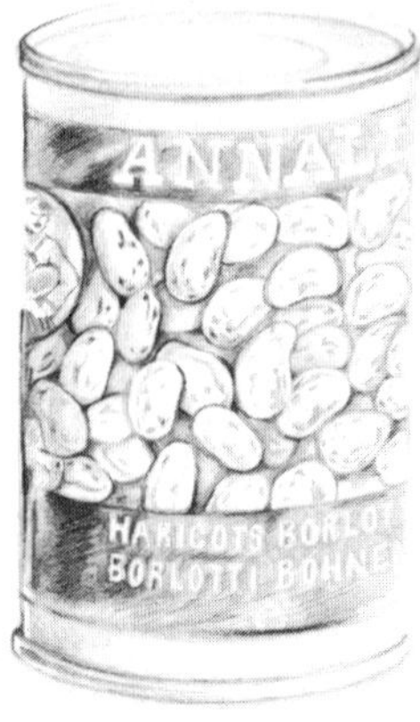

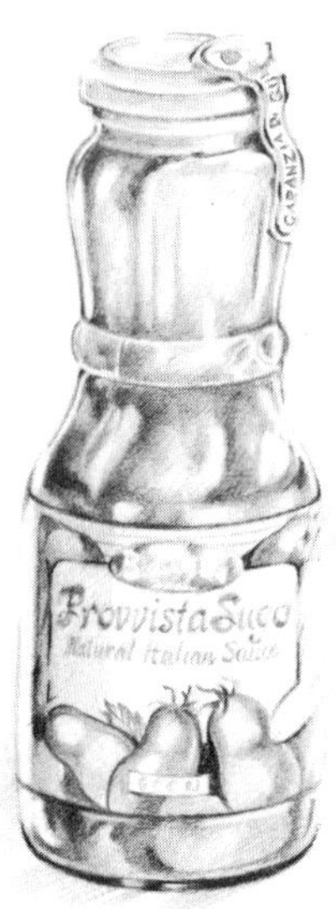

- Pulses, such as lentils, split peas and all sorts of dried beans, as well as canned pulses (for example, red beans, cannellini beans, borlotti beans, lentils, chick peas), which require much less time to cook than dried beans.
- Nuts, such as almonds, pine nuts, walnuts, and seeds, such as sesame, sunflower and pepita seeds.
- Spices of your choice can include curry powder, cummin seeds and powder, coriander seeds and powder, fennel seeds, chilli powder, paprika, prepared mustard, saffron, cinnamon sticks and ground cinnamon, vanilla essence and vanilla pods.
- Oils, such as olive oil, peanut oil, polyunsaturated oil and sesame oil, and a choice of vinegars.
- Canned fish, such as tuna and salmon, canned vegetables, such as corn and tomatoes, and canned fruits in natural juice, such as peaches, apricots and pears.

IN THE FREEZER

A couple of loaves of bread, some frozen peas or corn, home-made tomato sauce, chicken stock and chicken bones to make stock, and a few precooked well-labelled dishes for emergencies. I choose not to use the freezer extensively as fresh food tastes better but, of course, not everyone has the choice.

IN THE REFRIGERATOR

Apart from fresh vegetables and meats, we like to keep permanently on hand low-fat dairy products, such as milk, yoghurt and cheese, as well as bottled Italian tomato sauce, some eggs, fruit juices and mineral water.

We keep a large selection of seasonal fruits in the fruit bowl in the kitchen from which the children are free to help themselves.

Thus, if you make sure that your kitchen is efficiently arranged, and that you have on hand a good supply of basic ingredients, you are well on the way to speedy cooking. The recipes in this book will certainly make it easy for you to produce good food fast.

Fresh, light – and fast!
A stunning Thai soup of
prawns and noodles spiked
with chillies and coriander
(page 52)

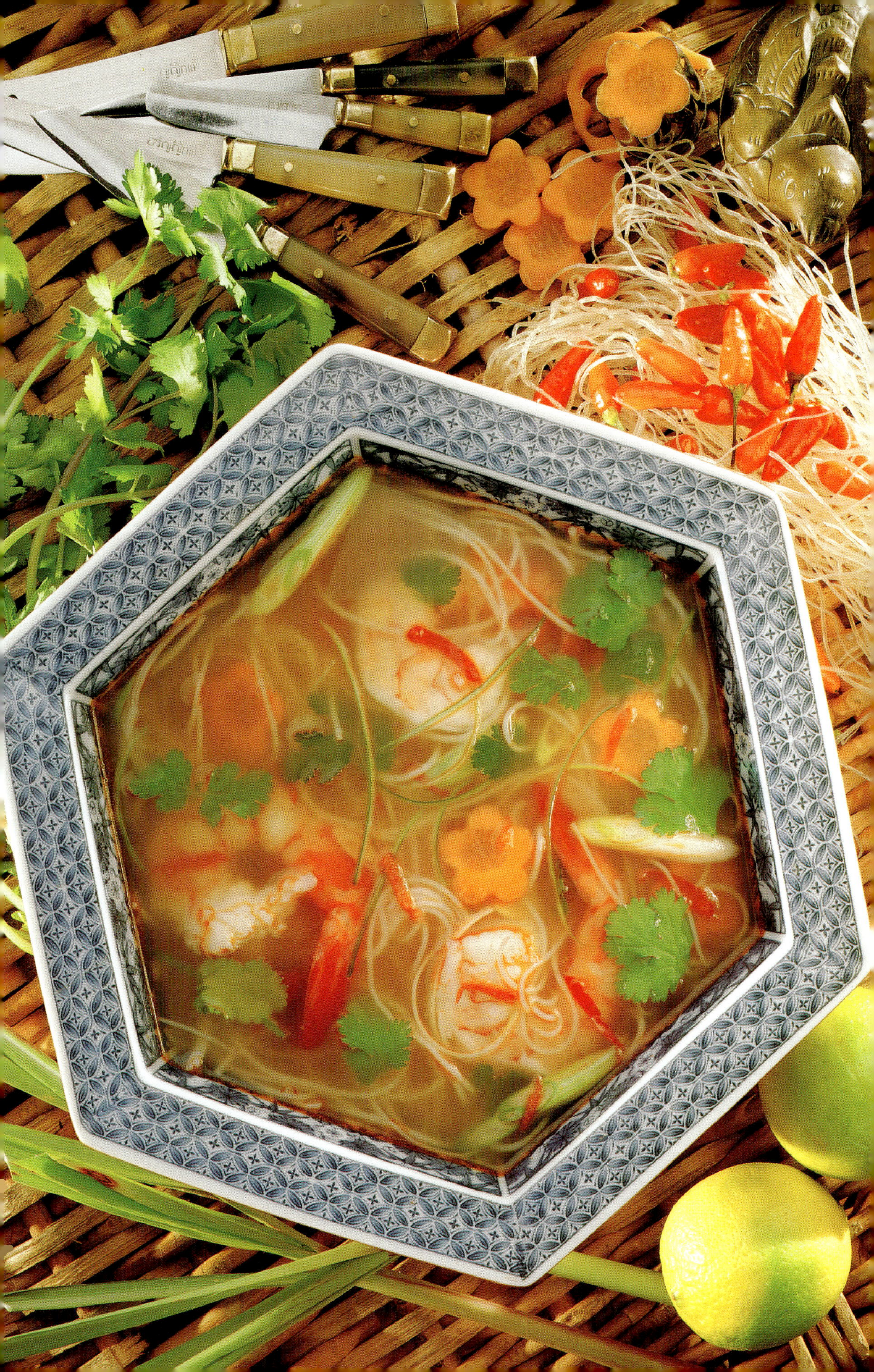

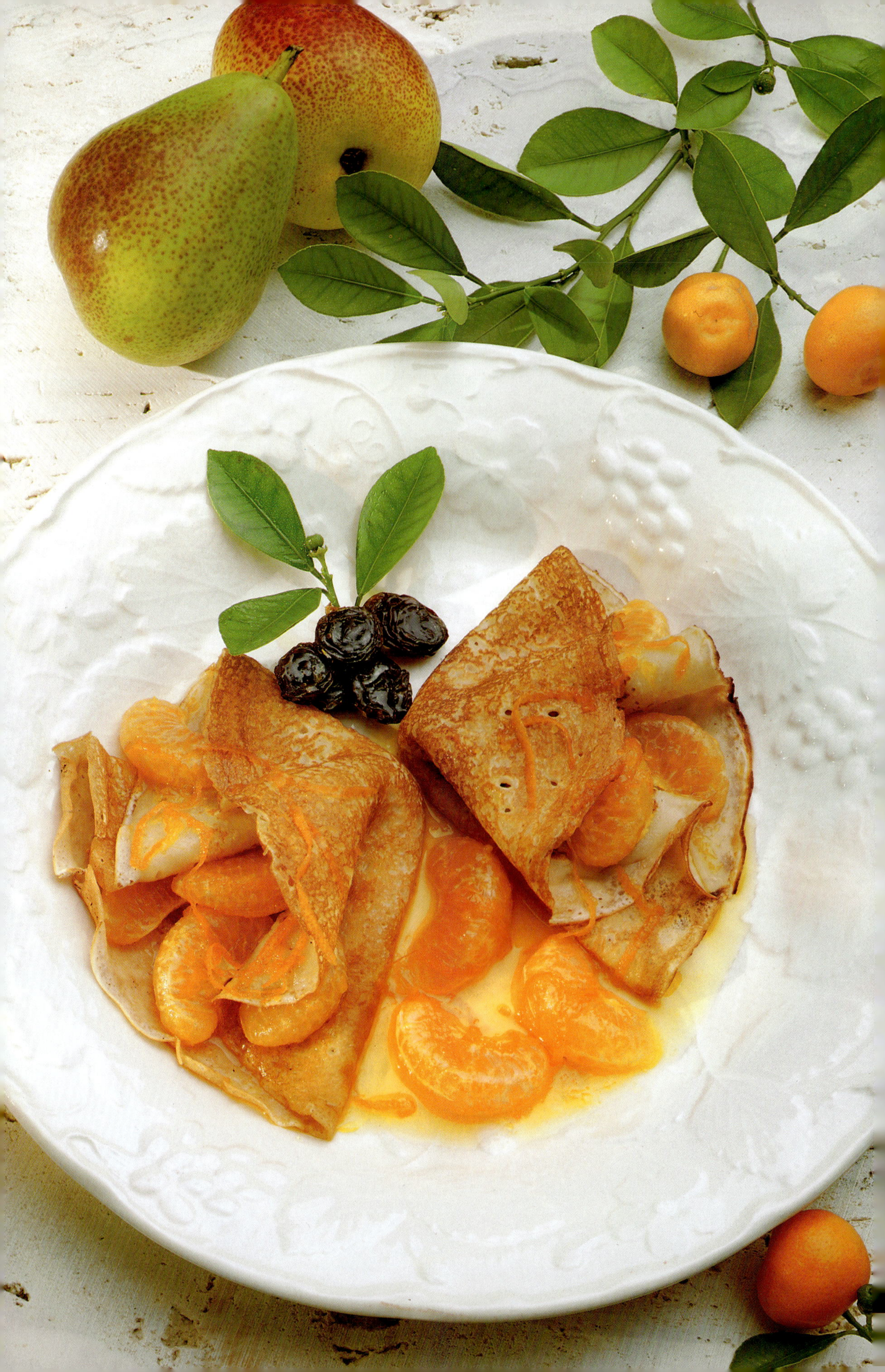

A Nine-week Cookery Course

So you dream of being a great cook? Cease dreaming and make your dream come true! Each of us has the potential to become a competent, happy cook – and therefore a fast cook. Certainly, some people are luckier than others, in that they were introduced as children or adolescents to the basics and joys of cooking by their parents or teachers. Others missed out altogether and lived in blissful ignorance until hit with the shock of having to cook by necessity.

I have designed this short course for people who have had little or no cookery experience and who have to cook. To begin and complete any course calls for some commitment, but a concerted effort will bring great satisfaction, for cooking is a source of many joys. The nine-week course will take you through the preparation of fifteen simple and varied dishes. You will learn to choose ingredients carefully and you will become familiar with basic cookery utensils and techniques. Furthermore, the course will introduce you to healthy cooking guidelines.

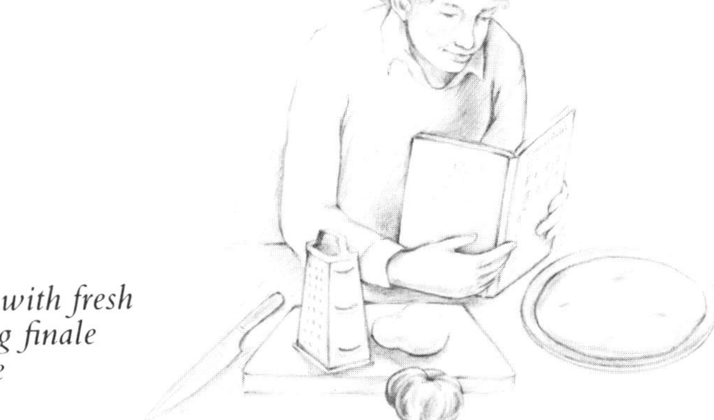

◁

Lacy thin pancakes with fresh mandarins – a fitting finale and family favourite (page 132)

Over the nine weeks of the course, the cook is asked to prepare each of the fifteen dishes three times. This method of practising a dish several times within a short period allows you to learn and remember the steps and important points that you may forget if preparing the dishes only once. You will also learn to prepare these dishes quickly. It may be that some of the recipes suggested are not quite to your taste. If so, just replace them with a similar recipe from the same chapter of the book. For instance, substitute a soup with another soup.

As you become familiar with each dish in the course, adapt it to your own taste if you wish. My recipes are only meant to guide you. Once you have mastered a dish, there is no need to follow it rigidly, and by ultimately experimenting with ingredients, your cooking will reflect your own personality. Have faith in yourself; don't be afraid of small failures, for you will learn greatly from them. In the words of Shakespeare, 'Nothing comes from doing nothing'.

Before we start our course it is necessary for you to read the basic information in the following pages. The chapter introductions also cover topics of vital interest to the inexperienced cook.

Cookware

Knives and pots and pans are expensive so young cooks inevitably own little cookware. This cooking course has been devised with that in mind, so the recipes are simple and use everyday cooking equipment. As you become a better cook, you will appreciate the help that the right equipment can give you in the kitchen and won't regret investing in what you need. Listed below is the equipment you will need over the nine weeks of this cookery course. If you cannot afford to buy some of the suggested items, borrow them. I have practised 'the borrowing method' for many years and believe that if we do it with books, we can do it with saucepans, too!

Knives

Knives are a cook's most important tool. Knives are to cooking what the racquet is to tennis. If you can afford only one knife, buy a medium-sized one with a blade about 15 cm (6 in) long. There are three basic knives that cover most cutting jobs. A small paring knife with a blade about 10 cm (4 in) long is ideal for peeling and trimming fruit and vegetables and for doing other small jobs. A medium to long knife with a wide, 20 cm (8 in) long blade is perfect for cutting vegetables into various shapes and for cutting some types of meat.

It takes fifteen seconds to sharpen a knife with a steel. Then cutting is a breeze.

A boning knife with a thin but strong blade about 15 cm (6 in) long trims fat from meat, portions chicken, and cuts small pieces of meat. To keep these knives sharp, you need a sharpening steel. For cutting bread and other foods, a serrated knife is most useful. The knives referred to as 'chefs' knives' are usually the best and are to be found in department stores and specialist cookware shops.

Saucepans

In this course you will need three different-sized saucepans: a small 1-litre saucepan, a medium 2-litre saucepan and a large saucepan that holds at least 4 litres. Choose the best quality you can afford and avoid aluminium saucepans. Food cooks better in stainless-steel pans. Don't feel that you need a complete set of saucepans, as there are sizes you may never use. Buy them one by one, according to your needs.

Frying pan

The size of the frying pan you choose depends on how many people you usually cook for. Avoid aluminium and choose stainless steel, enamel or iron.

Steamer

What would I do without my steamer? It is the most useful piece of equipment for cooking plain vegetables and keeping them warm until you are ready to serve them. Choose a stainless-steel steamer with a base measurement of at least 20 cm (8 in). I like a large steamer that will steam vegetables for four and even hold a whole chicken or a small fish as well.

Baking dishes

You will find having two different-sized baking dishes very handy: a small one for occasions such as baking two apples or reheating a small quantity of rice, and a large one for dishes like the baked tandoori-style fish in this chapter. Select a heavy baking dish that can be used on top of the stove as well as in the oven.

Oven rack

An oven rack allows the heat to circulate more effectively around the food being roasted and, therefore, saves on cooking time. As the food does not come into contact with the cooking fat, which collects in the roasting dish, it is less fatty.

Buy small potatoes for baking and steaming. They cook faster than large ones.

Bowls

Two or three mixing bowls are necessary in any kitchen. I prefer using glass, terracotta or stainless-steel bowls, and I dislike the feel of plastic. If you select attractive bowls you can also use them for serving vegetables and fruit salads.

Wok

The Asian wok is one of my favourite cooking utensils because it really involves the cook and requires little exertion. Choose a thin, iron wok at least 30 cm (12 in) in diameter and one with a lid. Avoid aluminium and stainless-steel woks. To stir-fry efficiently, you also need a special flat metal spoon that usually comes with wok sets. Asian grocery stores sell reasonably priced woks.

Other essential items

- a brush to coat your pan with a small amount of oil, and for other small jobs
- a vegetable peeler
- a couple of wooden spoons for stirring and mixing
- an egg lifter or flat metal spatula for transferring fish and meat from pan to plate
- a pepper grinder
- a large colander for draining pasta, vegetables and rice
- an apple corer
- a salad spinner to dry your leafy greens so that the salad dressing coats the leaves more efficiently

Shopping

I must confess that I love shopping for food. I find the beauty of fruit and vegetables stimulating and inspiring, and after years of meeting the same shopkeepers two or three times a week, I come to look on them as friends. Shopkeepers are an inexhaustible source of information, especially those with many years of experience. I cannot encourage readers enough to communicate with their local shopkeepers. Don't be afraid to tell them what you intend doing with the food you buy. They might just have a little hint for you.

I prefer butchers and poulterers who offer service rather than those who simply provide meat that is precut and prepackaged. A good butcher will trim the meat for you and sell you just what you need. Greengrocers that still offer service are generally of a good standard, but I do prefer self-service shops where I can select exactly what I need. For instance,

Learn to use a wok. Stir-frying is one of the quickest and easiest of cooking methods.

Really fresh, young vegetables have the sweetest flavour and cook the most quickly.

sometimes I may want small onions, or large bananas that will be ripe in two days' time. Choose your fruit and vegetables one by one and handle the food very gently. Take your time, look for spots or blemishes, and smell the fruit to see if it is ripe.

When organising the ingredients for any of the dishes in this course, you will find it easier and more efficient to make two detailed shopping lists – one for grocery items and one for fresh, perishable foods. Store dry foods in airtight containers and, if necessary, label them, for some foods, such as chilli powder and paprika, look alike. For the sake of freshness it is best to shop for perishable foods, such as meat, fish and vegetables, two or three times a week. Fish and minced meat are the most perishable of all and need to be purchased on the day they are to be consumed. Avoid buying fish on Mondays, as on this day most fishmongers sell fish left over from the weekend. Store fish on the top shelf of the refrigerator, where it is coldest. Minced meat and other meats are best stored in the meat tray of your refrigerator. Chicken pieces, lamb chops and casserole beef should be purchased no more than two days before you use them.

Most fruit and vegetables keep well for at least two or three days. Keep fruit in a bowl in the coolest part of the kitchen and store vegetables in the crisper at the bottom of the refrigerator. Avoid leaving food in a hot car for any length of time, and store ingredients in their right place as soon as you arrive home. The smell test is usually the surest way to assess the freshness of food. Your nose knows!

Being green in the kitchen

To save energy and water:
- cook just what you need and avoid overcooking food
- control the heat under boiling water and under the steamer
- preheat the oven for just the required amount of time and make sure that your oven, refrigerator and freezer doors close tightly and so are not losing energy
- microwave food when appropriate, as microwave ovens use less energy than gas and electric ovens
- put just enough water in the kettle and use suitable cooking utensils; for example, when cooking for one person use a small pan
- minimise the use of dishwashing machines as they consume large amounts of water and electricity

Take your own basket or carry bag when shopping to save paper and plastic bags.

Buy mineral water, soft drinks and wine in recyclable glass containers.

Growing your own vegetables, herbs and fruit will help to keep you, and the planet, healthy.

Cooking new dishes

Cooking a new dish is always a great challenge. It is something like walking in the dark. At first, there can be a sense of hopelessness but we soon gain confidence. To make the task a little easier, I have selected dishes that you may have eaten before or seen someone else cook.

Before doing your shopping, make a list of the ingredients you need to buy. At the same time, read the recipe thoroughly and, as you go, try to make a mental picture of the various steps and of the finished dish. Then, most importantly, allow yourself sufficient time to prepare the dish in a relaxed manner. If you feel hassled before starting the recipe, take a pause and sit down, take some deep breaths out in the garden, or drink a glass of water. Although I enjoy wine, I believe that drinking before cooking reduces the precision of my movements so I prefer to relax in other ways. The novelty of preparing a dish requires a clear mind and good concentration. Try to create a peaceful atmosphere with good lighting and avoid cooking with loud music or the television blaring. Clear a large working space, then read the recipe carefully and assemble the ingredients and equipment. You are now ready for the challenge.

Cooking is a bit like driving a car, for as you drive or cook you need to anticipate. The signs on the side of the road, or the suggested cooking times, are only guides. You are the one in control. The same journey or recipe never takes the same time – you don't go from point A to point B at the same speed every time. For instance, when frying food, you need to increase or reduce the heat according to what is happening in the pan. The food may be starting to burn or may not be cooking quickly enough. No cookbook can cover all the possible steps you will have to take. Any attempt to do so would result in very long, boring recipes.

You will take heart at your successes and learn enormously from your little failures and mistakes. No one is hopeless. You only fail if you give up trying, and practice makes a huge difference. I have burnt, undercooked and overcooked food and made my fair share of mess.

As you prepare food, clear up peelings and so on as you work, and place the food that is ready to be cooked on a clean plate, dish, tray or in a bowl, depending on what it is. Rinse dirty cookware and pile it neatly to make the washing up easier later on. When all the preparations are finished and the dish is cooking, avoid becoming involved in some other

When preparing salad ingredients, ask your children or partner to make the dressing.

If you make a double quantity of soup, you can freeze the extra to reheat for an instant meal.

activity that will distract you, unless of course it is quite safe to do so. This quiet cooking time is a good opportunity to take notes on the dish, and your observations will be of great help to you next time.

The end of the cooking is an important time and the challenge is in deciding when to stop the cooking. Basically, you need to rely on past experience and on the instructions provided in the recipe. The general rule is that food tastes better and is more nutritious when not overcooked. Also, food should be easy to chew. As you gain experience, you will work more quickly and be able to anticipate better, you will make more appropriate decisions and tire less, and you will enjoy cooking more and more. Art Linkletter said: 'Things turn out best for the people who make the best out of the way things turn out.'

The nine-week course

WEEK 1

At the start of the course, all the dishes you prepare will be new to you and I'm sure you will find the experience more enjoyable and less tiring if you are not too ambitious, satisfying yourself with cooking only one or two of the following dishes per day. They may be prepared in the order you choose.

To stir-fry vegetables quickly, cut them into small, regular pieces.

Vegetable soup (page 15)
Spaghetti with zucchini and pine nuts (page 16)
Ratatouille (page 17)
Fruit salad (page 18)
Hamburgers (page 18)

WEEK 2

Be sure to read the introduction to soups in chapter 5. This week, in addition to one new recipe, you will be preparing four dishes that you cooked last week. The cutting of vegetables should be coming more easily to you now and you will probably be able to work more quickly. Don't hesitate to adapt the dishes to your taste, but remember to use fat, salt and sugar in moderation. The new dish this week is a simple fish preparation and before doing it, read the introduction to fish in chapter 8.

NEW RECIPE
   Pan-fried fish fillets (page 19)

Children love making fruit
salads. Let them help save
you time.

REPEAT RECIPES
Vegetable soup (page 15)
Ratatouille (page 17)
Fruit salad (page 18)
Hamburgers (page 18)

WEEK 3

Read the introduction to pasta in chapter 6, to salads in
chapter 4 and to salad dressings in chapter 7. This
week you will be introduced to wok cooking and I
hope you will enjoy it as much as I do. By
concentrating on what is happening in the wok you'll
soon master the technique, which is one of the quickest
of all cooking techniques. With practice, you will be
able to prepare delicious, healthy stir-fry dishes. I
doubt that you'll have any problem with the two other
new dishes this week.

NEW RECIPES
Mixed salad with egg (page 19)
Pan-fried lamb chops with steamed beans and boiled
potatoes (page 20)
Stir-fried chicken with broccoli and bean sprouts
(page 21)

REPEAT RECIPES
Spaghetti with zucchini and pine nuts (page 16)
Pan-fried fish fillets (page 19)

WEEK 4

Read the introduction to pulses in chapter 6 and to
seasonings in chapter 7. Seasoning plays a very
important role in cooking, as you will find out when
you prepare the spicy dish of beans this week. At the
end of this week, you'll be an expert in cooking
spaghetti and in pan-frying fish. This week's dessert,
caramelised baked apple, is simple yet fun to make and
delicious.

NEW RECIPES
Caramelised baked apple (page 22)
Spicy vegetable and bean stew (page 23)

REPEAT RECIPES
Spaghetti with zucchini and pine nuts (page 16)
Stir-fried chicken with broccoli and bean sprouts
(page 21)
Pan-fried fish fillets (page 19)

You will always be able to
produce a quick meal if you
keep pasta, rice and pulses
permanently on hand.

WEEK 5

Read the introduction to rice in chapter 6 and to desserts in chapter 11. May I suggest that over the next few days you try to visit a major food market in your town or State. Look at the colours and enjoy the aromas. Be curious. This week you will cook the vegetable soup for the third time, and you could perhaps try it without referring to the recipe. If you wish, use different vegetables from those listed, and try the dish of lamb chops using vegetables of your choice this time. The new fish recipe is easy to prepare and the result is beautiful. Reread the introduction to fish in chapter 8 if you have time.

NEW RECIPES

  Baked tandoori-style fish (page 24)

  Rice with vegetables and parmesan cheese (page 24)

REPEAT RECIPES

  Vegetable soup (page 15)

  Pan-fried lamb chops with steamed beans and boiled potatoes (page 20)

  Spicy vegetable and bean stew (page 23)

WEEK 6

A well-sharpened boning knife is the most efficient for paring and deboning meat.

Read the introduction to meat in chapter 10. This will be the third time that you will have prepared stir-fried chicken and you must have learnt a lot from your experience, so you should now be ready to try other stir-fried dishes in this book. If you have access to fresh herbs, try adding a little finely sliced basil or tarragon or a pinch of curry powder, instead of lemon thyme, to the ratatouille. The new beef dish is simple but allow yourself sufficient time for the cooking, as it is the longest dish of the course.

NEW RECIPE

  Beef and vegetable casserole (page 25)

REPEAT RECIPES

  Ratatouille (page 17)

  Caramelised baked apple (page 22)

  Stir-fried chicken with broccoli and bean sprouts (page 21)

  Baked tandoori-style fish (page 24)

WEEK 7

Read the introduction to poultry in chapter 9. The chicken curry that you will prepare this week is the last new dish of the course. At home we cook this dish regularly. After your experience of preparing the spicy bean casserole and the baked tandoori-style fish you must be starting to understand a little more about the flavour of spices and will undoubtedly enjoy reading the introduction to seasonings in chapter 7. Again, don't hesitate to vary the vegetables used in the rice dish and the lamb chop recipe, trying vegetables you have not cooked before, if possible.

NEW RECIPE

Chicken and vegetable curry (page 26)

REPEAT RECIPES

Mixed salad with egg (page 19)

Pan-fried lamb chops with steamed beans and boiled potatoes (page 20)

Baked tandoori-style fish (page 24)

Rice with vegetables and parmesan cheese (page 24)

WEEK 8

Start by reading the introduction to vegetables in chapter 3. As there are no new recipes this week, you will enjoy the luxury of doing dishes you already know well. It may now be a good opportunity to try putting together a meal. For example, you might cook some plain rice to go with the chicken curry, make a salad to follow the spicy vegetable and bean casserole, or cook a special vegetable dish to accompany hamburgers.

REPEAT RECIPES

Hamburgers (page 18)

Caramelised baked apple (page 22)

Spicy vegetable and bean stew (page 23)

Beef and vegetable casserole (page 25)

Chicken and vegetable curry (page 26)

WEEK 9

This is the final week! I trust you have enjoyed the selection of dishes and dare I hope that some may even become your all-time favourites? After trying this week's five dishes, you will be ready to plan your own cookery evolution. It is important to keep cooking new dishes regularly and to adhere to the method of practising the same dishes several times over two or three weeks until you feel you have mastered them. Varying what you cook will help stimulate your interest in cooking and you might consider joining a cooking class, where you can observe an expert cooking right in front of you. Cookery schools and classes are listed in the *Yellow Pages*.

For a change from beef, think of making chicken or turkey burgers.

REPEAT RECIPES

Fruit salad (page 18)

Mixed salad with egg (page 19)

Rice with vegetables and parmesan cheese (page 24)

Beef and vegetable casserole (page 25)

Chicken and vegetable curry (page 26)

Now that you are no longer a beginner, cooking will become easier, faster and more enjoyable. Congratulations on completing this course!

Happy cooking.

Vegetable soup

A good vegetable soup is obtained by cooking a variety of vegetables that have contrasting flavour, texture and colour. Try to cut the vegetables in regular pieces so they will cook evenly, but don't worry if your slicing is inconsistent at first. Raw vegetables are some of the hardest ingredients of all and you will find it easier to cut them using a large knife. When familiar with making this soup, try creating your own combination of vegetables. The first time you make the soup, allow yourself about 35 mins, and, if cooking just for yourself, you may wish to freeze half of it once it is cold. Using canned corn will save time. Vegetable-cutting techniques for this soup and other recipes are shown on page 17.

SERVES 4

1 medium leek

1 medium carrot

½ stick celery

1 cob of corn

1 tsp olive oil

1 large potato

about ¼ cup parsley

freshly ground black pepper

Trim off any damaged leek leaves, and cut off and discard about one-third of the green part of the leek. Cut leek in four lengthwise, leaving the root intact, and wash thoroughly in lukewarm water to remove grit.

Peel carrot and cut in four lengthwise.

If celery is not tender, peel the stringy side then halve celery lengthwise.

Cut leek, carrot and celery into small, regular pieces.

Remove leaves and hair of corn and, using a short, sharp knife, remove kernels from cob.

Brush a large saucepan with oil and on low heat fry leek, carrot and celery for about 5 mins, stirring continuously with a wooden spoon. Add cold water to approximately 2 cm (¾ in) above the level of the vegetables, bring to boil and boil for 5 mins.

Meanwhile, peel and wash potato. Cut potato into about 1 cm (⅓ in) thick slices then into about 1 cm (⅓ in) wide sticks, and dice. Add diced potato and corn kernels to soup and boil rapidly for about 10 mins or until potato is soft.

Meanwhile, wash and chop parsley. Stir chopped parsley into soup and season with a little pepper just before serving.

Spaghetti with zucchini and pine nuts

Always cook pasta in a large quantity of lightly salted boiling water and follow the cooking instructions that are usually printed on the pack. If you wish, you can use another type of pasta for this dish. Zucchini is one of the softest vegetables and you will enjoy practising your dicing with it. This dish is delicious for its contrast of textures. Buy a piece of fresh parmesan and grate it yourself. Allow about 30 mins for this dish.

SERVES 1

¼ **small onion**

1 medium tomato

2 small zucchini

1 sprig parsley

½ **clove garlic**

1 tsp olive oil

100 g (3½ oz) spaghetti, wholemeal or other

1 tbsp pine nuts

freshly ground black pepper

1 tbsp grated parmesan cheese

Peel and chop onion.

Wash and dice tomato.

Wash zucchini and trim ends. Dice zucchini.

Wash parsley and slice finely.

Crush garlic, remove skin and chop finely.

Bring to the boil a medium saucepan three-quarters full of lightly salted water.

Meanwhile, heat olive oil in a small saucepan and, using a wooden spoon, gently stir-fry onion for about 1 min. Add zucchini, stir for another minute and add tomato. Bring to boil and cook on high heat for 2 mins. Turn off heat and put aside.

Add spaghetti to boiling water and when all the spaghetti sinks, stir briefly to prevent it from sticking together. Cooking time varies depending on the type of spaghetti you use. Check the cooking by testing one strand of spaghetti. The easiest way is to remove it using a fork, then to cool it under the tap. Bite into it. The spaghetti should be firm but tender. If the centre is still a little dry, cook the spaghetti a bit longer and test again. Drain spaghetti in a colander and shake colander to extract all the water. Return spaghetti to saucepan and gently stir in vegetables, parsley, garlic and pine nuts. Season with a little black pepper and reheat gently for 30 secs.

Serve sprinkled with a little grated parmesan.

Ratatouille

Ratatouille is a Mediterranean preparation of mixed vegetables and always includes tomatoes. Making this dish provides practice in cutting vegetables and those listed below are available at most times of the year. Try growing a few different herbs in pots or in your garden. You will find herbs at most nurseries. Alternatively, use dried herbs, but the flavour is not as good. Ratatouille can be eaten on its own with grated cheese and bread and is even delicious cold, or you can serve it with pan-fried fish or meat, with a roast or with pasta. Allow 30 mins from beginning to end for this dish.

SERVES ABOUT 3

1 small brown onion

2 cloves garlic

1 red or green capsicum

1 zucchini

1 small eggplant

3 tomatoes

½–1 tbsp olive oil

1 sprig lemon thyme

freshly ground black pepper

Peel and halve onion and cut into approximately 1 cm (⅓ in) squares. Using a large knife, crush garlic cloves and discard peel.

As you cut all the following ingredients, arrange them in separate piles.

Halve capsicum and remove seeds.

Trim ends of zucchini and eggplant.

Wash capsicum, zucchini, eggplant and tomatoes in cold water. Cut all vegetables into pieces that are a little smaller than bite-size.

Heat oil in a medium saucepan and, using a wooden spoon, stir-fry onion for 2 mins on medium heat. Add garlic and capsicum and fry for another 2 mins. Reduce heat slightly if vegetables start browning. Add zucchini, eggplant, tomato and thyme, and season with a little pepper. Stir to mix vegetables well. Cover pan and cook on medium heat for about 15 mins.

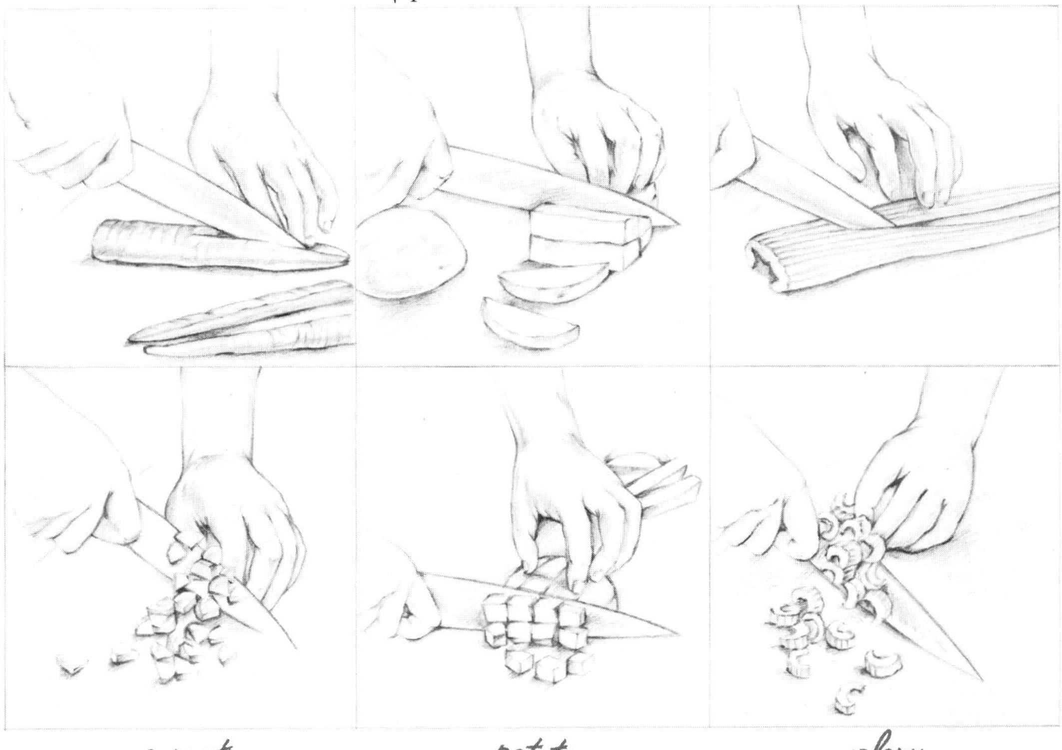

carrot   potato   celery

Fruit salad

An interesting fruit salad should be one of the basics for the busy cook. The secret of a good fruit salad is to use a selection of just-ripened fruits of varying texture. You need to add a flavoursome liquid and I like freshly squeezed orange juice for most fruit salads. Try preparing the following recipe two or three times within the next two weeks and then create your own concoction using seasonal fruits. Additional sugar is not usually necessary. Once you have assembled your ingredients, allow 15 mins for the preparation.

SERVES ABOUT 2

1 orange
1 ripe pear
1 banana
1 kiwi fruit
8 raw almonds
1 tsp sugar (optional)

Squeeze orange and place juice in a medium bowl.

Wash, quarter and core pear and cut into 5 mm (¼ in) slices, adding them directly to bowl. Stir pear gently to cover with juice.

Peel banana, cut into similar slices and add to bowl.

Peel and quarter kiwi fruit and slice similarly. Add to bowl and stir gently.

Using a large knife and a chopping board, cut almonds into small pieces and add to bowl just before serving.

If not serving your fruit salad within 15 mins, cover and refrigerate.

Hamburgers

Hamburgers can be made using all types of minced meat. Ask your butcher for lean mince and remember that about 125 g (¼ lb) per person is sufficient. For the hamburgers to hold well together, the ingredients must be very well mixed. You may enjoy serving your hamburgers in the traditional way, that is, in a roll with mixed raw vegetables like carrot, lettuce, celery and tomatoes. It makes a nutritious, light meal. The first time you prepare this dish, allow about 25 mins for preparation and cooking, but after a few times you will find that you can make it without even referring to the recipe.

MAKES 1 HAMBURGER

1 sprig parsley
125 g (¼ lb) lean minced beef or other lean minced meat
2 tbsp cold water
1 tbsp dried breadcrumbs
a pinch of curry powder
1 tsp chopped onion
freshly ground black pepper
a little olive, peanut or polyunsaturated oil

Wash and chop parsley.

In a bowl and using your fingers, thoroughly mix mince, water, breadcrumbs, curry powder, onion, parsley and a little pepper. Form mixture into a hamburger shape about 2 cm (¾ in) thick.

Brush a small frying pan with oil. Heat pan and cook hamburger on medium heat, adjusting temperature if necessary. It is best not to push or move the meat as it cooks. Turn hamburger halfway through and, depending on how you like your meat, cook for 3 to 5 mins on each side. Check the cooking by pressing the meat with your finger. If very soft, it is not cooked inside. If dry and inflexible to the touch, it is well done. The ideal for my taste is when the meat is firm but still a little flexible.

Serve immediately.

Pan-fried fish fillets

A fish dish is difficult to plan ahead because one never knows what varieties of fish will be available. At your fishmonger's, take a good look at what is on offer and ask for advice. Observe the shoppers who appear confident and see what they buy. It is best to choose a whole fish and ask for it to be scaled and filleted on the spot. Or select a moist but firm-looking fillet. If you plan to serve the fish with vegetables, start preparing the vegetables before cooking the fish. Allow about 15 mins to prepare and cook this dish.

SERVES 1

1 tbsp plain flour

a 150 g (5 oz) piece of fish fillet

freshly ground black pepper

a little olive oil

1 lemon wedge

Sprinkle flour on a plate. Coat fish fillet on all sides with flour and season it with a little pepper.

Brush a small frying pan with a little oil. When pan is hot, carefully place fillet in pan with the skinless side facing down. Without moving fish, cook the first side for 2 to 4 mins, depending on thickness of fillet. Turn fish over and cook the second side for 2 to 4 mins. The fish changes colour during cooking and is ready when the flesh flakes easily and when you can probe it with the blade of a small knife without meeting any resistance. Squeeze lemon juice on fish and serve.

Mixed salad with egg

The secret of a good salad lies in achieving a pleasant contrast of textures. The dressing, which contains fat, must be kept to a minimum and the green leaves need to be well dried so that the dressing coats well and so fulfils its role. Once you have assembled all your ingredients, allow about 20 mins to prepare this salad. For a one-dish meal, add tuna, olives and anchovies to make salad niçoise, and serve with crusty bread.

SERVES ABOUT 2

2 eggs

about 6 lettuce leaves

1 medium carrot

2 walnuts

½ green capsicum

½ tsp red wine vinegar

freshly ground black pepper

¼ tsp mustard

2 tsp peanut or polyunsaturated oil

Bring a small saucepan three-quarters full of water to the boil. Using a spoon, gently lower eggs into water, return water to boil, reduce to a simmer and cook eggs for 9 mins. Remove eggs from water and place in cold water to cool.

Meanwhile, wash lettuce leaves in a large quantity of cold water then drain. If you have a salad spinner, dry lettuce leaves in it. Otherwise, shake them gently. Tear leaves into two or three pieces.

Peel carrot and grate finely. Break walnut shells and remove walnut meat. Cut it into small pieces.

Remove capsicum seeds. Wash capsicum and slice thinly.

In a salad bowl, thoroughly mix vinegar with a little pepper and mustard, then stir in oil. Add grated carrot, walnut, capsicum and lettuce leaves and toss gently.

Carefully peel eggs and cut into quarters. Place attractively on top of salad.

Pan-fried lamb chops with steamed beans and boiled potatoes

Preparing this dish is a good way of learning about timing when cooking the various ingredients that compose a meal, and, of course, the vegetables and meat need to be ready at the same time. Of the three main ingredients used in this recipe, the potatoes are the least fragile and so are cooked first. Steaming vegetables is an excellent technique because, once ready, they can be kept warm for a little while in the uncovered steamer with no risk of their being overcooked. If you wish, the chops can be replaced by 150 g (5 oz) steak. If preparing this dish for more than one person, simply increase the ingredients accordingly and use larger pans; the cooking time will be about the same. Once you have assembled your ingredients allow about 30 mins for the preparation. With a little practice you will need less time. Start by reading the recipe carefully.

SERVES 1

2 or 3 small potatoes

150 g (5 oz) French beans

2 loin lamb chops

a little olive oil

freshly ground black pepper

1 lemon wedge

Wash potatoes in lukewarm water. Place in a small saucepan and cover with cold water. Bring water to boil. Cook potatoes for 10 to 15 mins, depending on their size.

Meanwhile, top and tail beans.

Using a sharp knife, trim and discard all visible fat from chops.

Bring about 2 cups of water to boil in steamer. Place beans in top compartment, cover and cook for 6 to 10 mins.

Meanwhile, brush frying pan with a little olive oil and place on medium to high heat. When you see the oil becoming hot, add chops to pan. Refrain from moving or pricking chops, and cook the first side for 3 to 5 mins. Turn chops and cook the second side for 3 to 5 mins, reducing heat if you think it is too high.

While cooking chops, check potatoes by piercing them with the blade of a small knife. They are cooked when the knife goes through easily. Turn off heat, drain potatoes and keep them in covered saucepan.

At the same time check the beans. Take one bean with a fork, cool it under the tap and taste it. If it is hard to break with your teeth, cook beans a little more, but if tender though still a little firm, the beans are ready. Turn off heat under steamer and remove lid.

Check the cooking of chops by pressing the meat with your finger. If very soft, the meat is not cooked inside. If it feels dry and inflexible to the touch, it is overcooked. If the meat is firm but still a little flexible, it is ideally cooked. Turn off heat, season chops with a little freshly ground black pepper and cover with a lid or foil for 1 min. Meanwhile, serve potatoes and beans on plate, then chops with any pan juices. Serve with a wedge of lemon.

▷

A fast fruit finish – golden peaches and red berries in a luscious summer dessert (page 129)

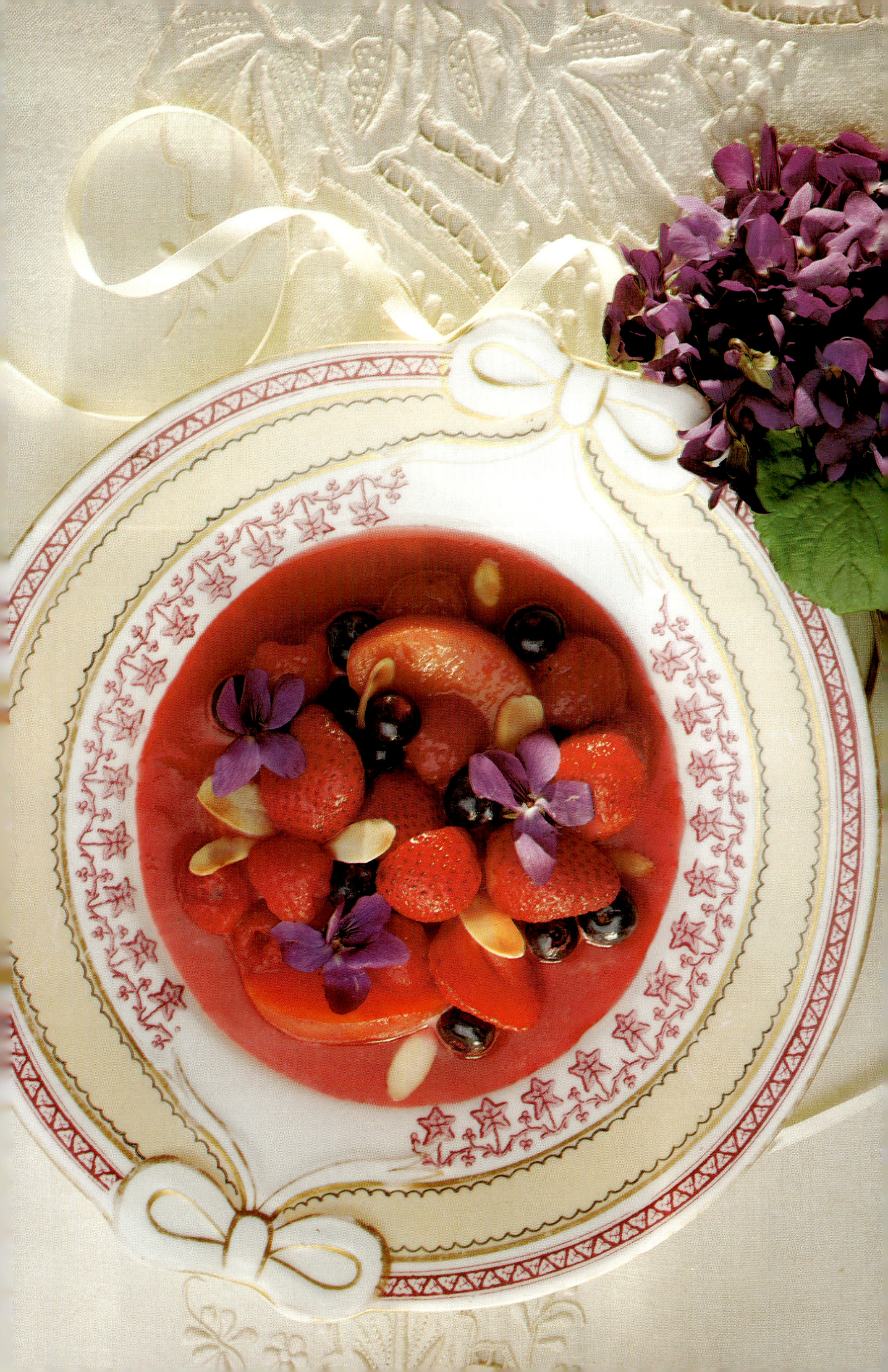

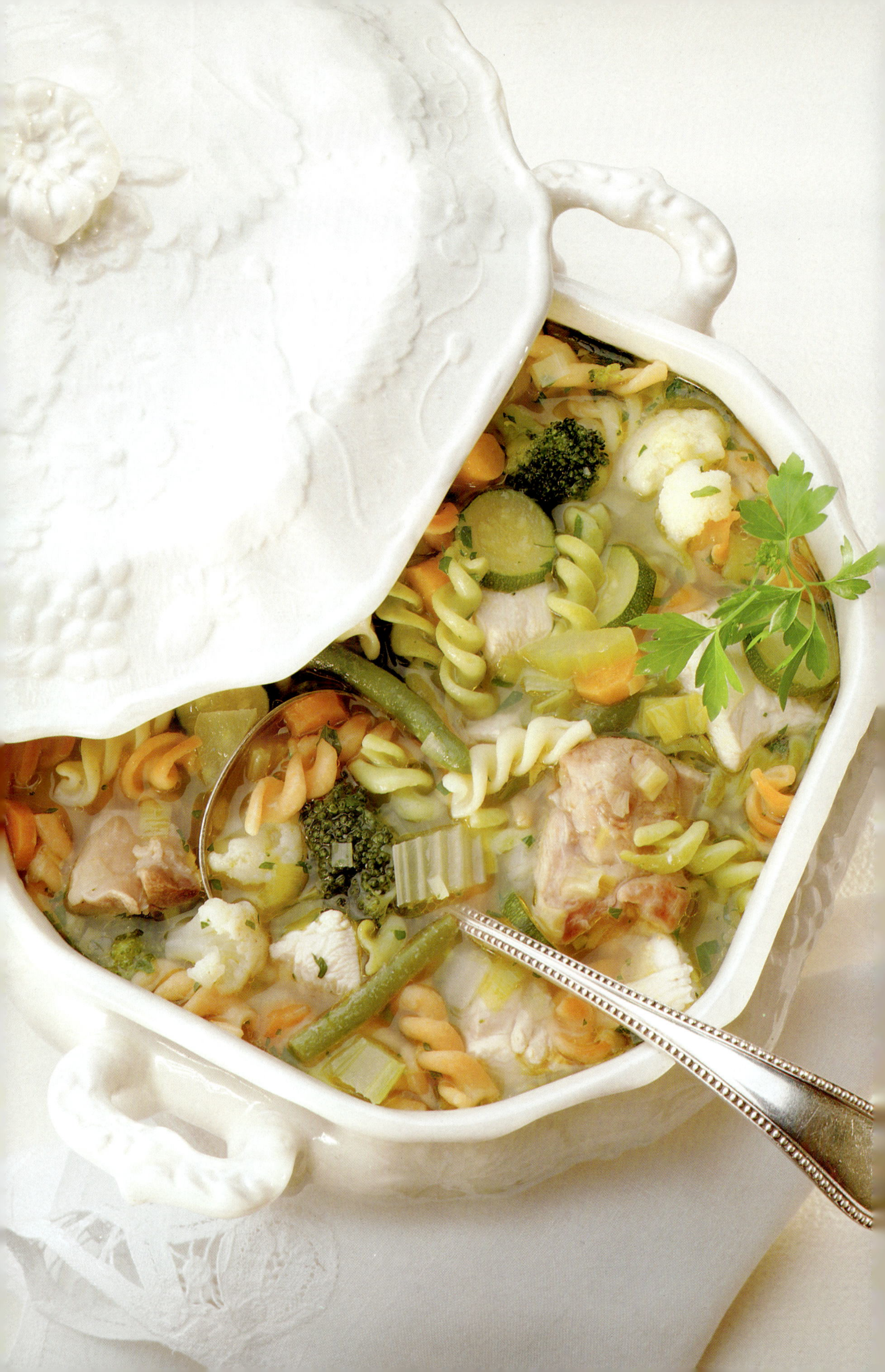

Stir-fried chicken with broccoli and bean sprouts

The wok is one of my favourite cooking utensils. Its large heating surface seals food rapidly, so stir-frying is a fast and economical way of cooking. Ingredients cooked in a wok must be cut into bite-size pieces or even smaller, and before use, the wok needs to be very clean. Heat the wok before adding any oil, and remember that the contents of the wok need to be stirred constantly to prevent the food from sticking and burning. After a few attempts, you will enjoy cooking with a wok. Allow about 30 mins to prepare and cook this dish.

SERVES 1

1 chicken fillet

1 tsp salt-reduced soy sauce

1 tsp lemon juice

½ tsp cornflour

150 g (5 oz) broccoli

about ½ cup bean sprouts

½ clove garlic

½ tbsp peanut or polyunsaturated oil

¼ cup water

freshly ground black pepper

Remove skin of chicken and discard it. Cut chicken into approximately 1 cm (1/3 in) thick strips. In a bowl stir chicken with soy sauce, lemon juice and cornflour.

Wash broccoli. Cut broccoli into flowerets and then into bite-size pieces, cutting stalks diagonally.

Wash bean sprouts and drain well.

Crush garlic using the blade of a large knife then peel garlic.

Heat wok for a few seconds then heat oil in wok. When hot, add garlic and chicken pieces and stir-fry on high heat until all the chicken pieces change colour. This takes about 1 min. Transfer chicken to a plate. Add broccoli to wok and stir-fry for a few seconds before adding water down the inside of the wok. Cover wok and cook for 1 min. Remove lid, add bean sprouts and stir-fry until broccoli and bean sprouts are soft. Mix chicken with vegetables and stir well for about 1 min. Season with a little pepper and serve.

◁

Chunky chicken and vegetable soup with pasta — a speedy, one-dish midweek meal (page 57)

Caramelised baked apple

You have probably already enjoyed this dessert at some time or another. The dish can be prepared a little in advance or may be cooked as you are eating your meal. Choose regular-sized, unblemished apples and look for a pleasant, sweet apple smell which indicates good flavour. A yellowish tinge means the apple is ripe. I enjoy Granny Smiths best but other apples are also suitable. If preparing this dish for more than two people, increase the ingredients proportionally. This only takes about 15 mins to prepare. While it is baking – which takes about 45 mins – you can prepare the rest of the meal.

SERVES 2

2 medium apples
½ small banana
4 raw almonds
2 tbsp sultanas
4 tbsp water or apple juice
1 tsp sugar

Preheat oven to about 180°C/350°F.

Wash and gently core apples, using an apple corer or small knife. Check inside and remove any remaining pips. Using the same knife, make a shallow cut all around the apple at the centre. This helps prevent the skin from bursting during cooking.

Cut the half banana lengthwise into four pieces.

Cut almonds into several pieces.

Place apples in a small baking dish and fill them with banana, almonds and sultanas, placing any remaining filling around them. Spoon water over apples and sprinkle with sugar. Bake in the top part of the oven for about 45 mins then check the cooking by piercing apples with the blade of a small knife. If soft, they are ready. Don't worry if the apples collapse a little, for they will still taste delicious.

Using an oven mitt, remove dish from oven. Lift apples onto plates, spoon juice over them and serve.

Add a little cold water to baking dish to facilitate the washing up later.

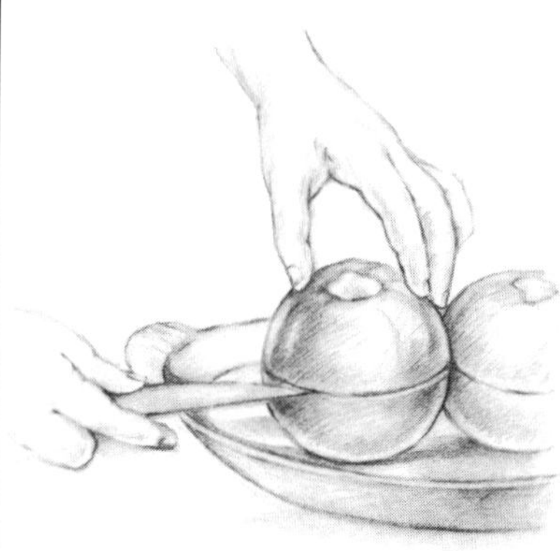

Spicy vegetable and bean stew

This recipe is not fast, but it is designed to introduce the beginner cook to an important technique. Most pulses need to be soaked overnight or for at least 12 hrs, but this is really no trouble at all. Simply measure the quantity needed and place in cold water. It only takes a minute or two. Pulses, that is, dried beans, lentils and chick peas, are delicious, satisfying and easy to prepare. Dried beans are available from supermarkets and health-food stores and there are many varieties. I suggest trying the white cannellini beans, which keep well for several months in the pantry. This is a vegetarian dish that you can adapt to your own taste by adding spices, herbs and vegetables of your choice. Once the beans have been soaked, allow about 20 mins for preparation and about 1 hr for cooking.

SERVES ABOUT 2

½ cup dried cannellini beans or other dried beans

2 tomatoes

1 clove garlic

1 medium carrot

1 green capsicum

2 sprigs parsley

½ tsp ground cummin

½ tsp curry powder

a pinch of chilli powder

Soak cannellini beans in a large quantity of cold water for at least 12 hrs.

Wash and quarter tomatoes.

Crush garlic using the blade of a large knife, then peel garlic.

Peel and slice carrot.

Halve capsicum and remove seeds. Wash and quarter each half.

Drain beans and discard water.

Place tomato, garlic, carrot, capsicum, parsley, cummin, curry powder, chilli powder and beans in a medium saucepan. Cover with cold water and bring to boil. Reduce heat to a simmer, cover pan and cook for 50 mins to 1 hr. The stew is ready when the beans are tender. The beans will absorb some of the water so make sure there is always a little water left in the bottom of the pan and add a little extra water, if necessary, during cooking.

SERVING SUGGESTION: This dish is delicious eaten with good wholegrain bread.

Baked tandoori-style fish

The preparation of this delicious dish will familiarise you with the technique of baking fish and with using spices. Ask your fishmonger for a very fresh fish weighing about 300 g (11 oz) and suitable for baking. Depending on the catch and where you live, different varieties will be available. Ask for the fish to be cleaned and scaled and for the fins to be cut off. If serving this dish with steamed vegetables, start cooking the vegetables before you cook the fish. Allow about 25 mins to prepare and cook this dish.

SERVES 1

1 whole fish weighing about 300 g (11 oz)

1 small piece of ginger

½ tsp curry powder

½ tsp paprika

a pinch of cayenne pepper

freshly ground black pepper

2 tsp low-fat natural yoghurt

1 tsp lemon juice

Rinse the insides of the fish, making sure there is no blood left. Pat fish dry with a towel and make about four shallow cuts across either side of the fish about 0.6 cm (¼ in) deep. This helps the fish cook evenly.

Preheat oven to 220°C/450°F.

Peel and grate about 1 tsp ginger.

In a small bowl combine ginger, curry powder, paprika, cayenne pepper, a little black pepper, yoghurt and lemon juice. Brush fish all over with this preparation and place fish on an oven rack set in a baking dish. Cook in preheated oven for about 12 mins. Using an egg lifter or long spatula, gently transfer fish to a plate.

Personally, I prefer to eat a whole fish on its own and then to enjoy some vegetables or other food as a second course.

Rice with vegetables and parmesan cheese

This is a satisfying light meal and rice can be cooked with many different kinds of vegetables, herbs and spices. Remember that brown rice is more nourishing than white rice and that long-grain rice takes less time to cook than short-grain rice because short-grain rice is fatter. In the interests of freshness, it is best to buy a piece of fresh parmesan and grate it yourself, though the pre-grated variety can be used for convenience. This dish can be prepared in advance then reheated in a low oven. Allow about 1 hr for this dish.

SERVES 2

½ brown onion

2 sticks celery

1 medium carrot

1 tsp olive oil

¾ cup long-grain brown rice

1¼ cups water

freshly ground black pepper

2–4 tbsp grated parmesan cheese

Peel and dice onion.

Wash and trim celery. Halve celery lengthwise then dice it. Peel and dice carrot.

Heat oil in a medium saucepan and, using a wooden spoon, stir in onion, celery and carrot. Fry gently for 3 to 4 mins but don't allow the vegetables to brown. Add rice and stir in well before adding water. Season with a little pepper and bring to boil. Reduce to a simmer, cover pan and cook for 35 to 40 mins. The rice is ready when it is tender and by that time the water will have been absorbed by the rice. If necessary, towards the end of the cooking, add a little hot water from the kettle.

Stir in grated cheese just before serving.

Beef and vegetable casserole

Of all the dishes in this course, this one takes the longest time because casserole beef should be tender and needs about 1¼ hrs to cook. I include this recipe because making a casserole is an essential skill for the cook. In fact it is not a difficult dish and you can easily prepare it in advance and reheat it when required. Ask your butcher for lean casserole meat. The use of wine is optional but gives the dish a beautiful flavour. Allow about 30 mins to prepare and 1¼ hrs to cook this dish.

SERVES ABOUT 2

about 350 g (12½ oz) lean casserole beef

½ brown onion

1 clove garlic

1 tomato

1 tbsp plain flour

a little peanut or polyunsaturated oil

¼ cup red wine (optional)

1 cup water

2 sprigs parsley

a small pinch of salt

freshly ground black pepper

2 carrots

1 medium potato

about ½ cup shelled peas

Trim meat of all fat and cut into approximately 3 cm (1½ in) cubes. Some pieces will inevitably be smaller than others.

Peel and slice onion.

Crush and peel garlic.

Wash tomato and cut into eight pieces.

In a small bowl, toss meat in a little flour to coat it.

Brush a medium saucepan with oil. Heat pan on high heat, add meat and, stirring with a wooden spoon, brown meat to seal it on all sides. Add onion, stir for 1 min then add tomato, wine, water, garlic and parsley. Season with salt and a little pepper. Bring to a simmer, cover and cook for 1 hr. Check the cooking two or three times, stirring gently to make sure it simmers well.

Meanwhile, peel carrots and potato and slice into bite-size pieces.

After the hour has elapsed, check the meat by tasting it. If it is almost tender, add carrot, potato and peas to saucepan, stir gently and cook for about 15 mins until potato and carrot are tender. If the meat is still a bit tough, cook a little longer before adding the vegetables.

Chicken and vegetable curry

You will enjoy this flavoursome curry, which is the most sophisticated dish of the course. This recipe introduces you to the many spices and seasonings available, which you can use in many quicker recipes. You will see that in a spicy dish each spice contributes its own flavour. For instance, cummin has a very aromatic, sweet flavour, while chilli is hot. Give yourself enough time for preparation and cooking, allowing about 1 hr in all once you have assembled the ingredients. If anything, a dish such as this improves if left for a little while, so it is ideal if you want to cook it when you have time and reheat it a little later.

SERVES ABOUT 4

about 200 g (7 oz) pumpkin

1 medium carrot

about ¼ cauliflower

2 tomatoes

4 chicken thighs

1 small brown onion

2 cloves garlic

a 2 cm (¾ in) piece of ginger

1 tbsp peanut oil

½ tsp cummin seeds

½ tsp fennel seeds

3 tsp curry powder

1½ cups water

1 tbsp desiccated coconut

½ tsp hot chilli paste (optional)

Cut pumpkin into bite-size pieces and peel it.

Peel carrot and cut into bite-size pieces.

Wash cauliflower and cut into bite-size flowerets.

Wash tomatoes and remove cores, using a paring knife. Dice tomatoes.

Skin chicken thighs and discard skin.

Peel onion and garlic and finely chop both.

Peel ginger and grate finely.

Place oil, onion, garlic, and ginger in a large saucepan. Add cummin and fennel seeds and on low heat gently fry for about 5 mins, stirring with a wooden spoon. Avoid browning. After 5 mins the onion will be a little transparent. Add curry powder and stir for 1 min before adding tomato. Bring to boil on high heat and boil for 2 mins. Stir in chicken thighs, pumpkin, carrot and water. Bring to a simmer, cover and cook for 10 mins.

Gently stir in cauliflower, cover again and cook for a further 10 mins.

Stir in desiccated coconut and chilli paste.

If the sauce is a little runny, gently boil the curry, uncovered, for a few minutes to reduce some of the liquid.

SERVING SUGGESTION: Serve with rice. If well organised, you might like to prepare a small platter of accompaniments such as lemon wedges, sliced banana and sultanas.

Vegetable Delights

Eat up your vegetables! They're good for you! This desperate plea is probably familiar to all parents of young children. Adults all over the world have grown to love vegetables. We know that eating a variety of the garden's delights provides fibre, vitamins and other good things that can help to protect against some cancers. Generally a diet that is high in a good variety of vegetables is correspondingly low in fat and energy (kilojoules) so in this way can also reduce the risk of heart disease and related illnesses. In a word, vegetables help to keep the body healthy.

Strangely enough, in most affluent countries of the world eating patterns are such that the role of vegetables is viewed as a secondary one. Vegetables are seen as a mere garnish to other foods rich in meat fat that we seem to find more attractive. Vegetables need to regain the high status they held for thousands of years but lost only a few decades ago. Their secondary position is perhaps best illustrated by the ludicrously small drawer allocated to them in most refrigerators. There is simply not enough room for a bunch of celery or a cabbage in the average vegetable crisper!

Today's leading nutritionists do not suggest that we all become vegetarian (although that is one choice, but it is important to understand that a nutritious vegetarian diet is not achieved simply by serving more vegetables in place of meat). Rather, they advise us to consume a greater variety and quantity of fresh vegetables.

The recipes in this chapter are ideal for those who are watching the clock as well as their health: well balanced, delicious, and on the table in minutes.

Kids and vegetables

Many mums and dads are concerned that their children do not eat a good variety of vegetables. When I was small I recall not being able to face the strong taste of leek and beetroot, yet now I love all vegetables. It is not uncommon for most children to take years to become familiar with and enjoy the textures and natural flavours of most vegetables. For a child, the experience of tasting a new vegetable is not unlike meeting a stranger for the first time. As humans we are naturally cautious when encountering the unknown. So even if parents tell a child that carrots are good, the untrained palate may find the flavour rather overwhelming at first bite. When you think of it, the flavour of a carrot is quite strong.

The child's first reaction might be surprise rather than rejection. No matter what, the brain of the child registers the flavour. Parents can try presenting a vegetable frequently over a period of time, without making a fuss or insisting that the child eat it. I noticed with interest that my elder son enjoyed grated carrot for years before he liked the vegetable cooked. Some children may enjoy a purée of carrot and not whole cooked carrots. As every parent knows, texture certainly plays an important role in the game of taste. To soften the strong flavour of a vegetable purée, mix in a little potato and the kids might just love it.

Introduce your children to as many different vegetables as you can, in sandwiches, soups, stir-fried dishes and pies. Roast, steam and microwave them. Above all, ask the children to help prepare vegetables. I'm convinced that this has a positive influence on eating habits. I have also found that the concept of the seasons fascinates children and encourages them to eat vegetables that are in season.

If a child persistently rejects all vegetables and fruits, advice can always be sought from a professional dietitian. Remember though, as children grow, so do their palates. So don't worry, Mum and Dad!

Fresh is best

The fresher vegetables are, the more beautiful they taste. Who could be better qualified to judge than those who grow their own vegetables? Most of us need to rely on the markets for our produce, however. We are advised to buy the more delicate vegetables, like all greens, cauliflower, bean sprouts, and so on, at least two or three times a week. Of course, they should be kept in the vegetable crisper of the refrigerator. Other

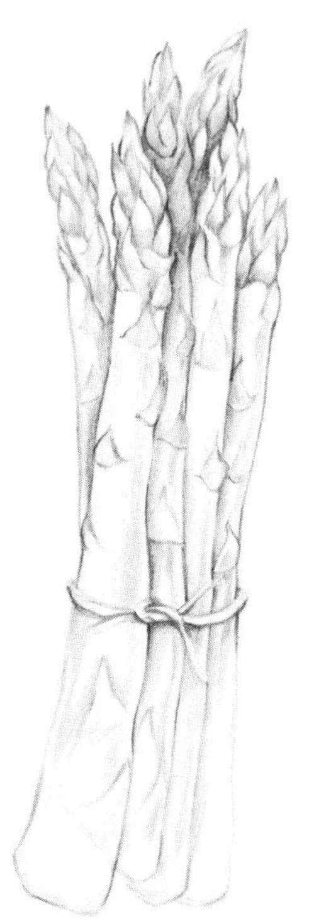

Salads made from raw vegetables are healthy and quick to prepare.

vegetables, such as onions, garlic, pumpkin and potatoes, can be purchased less frequently and stored in a cool, dry and preferably dark place. Tomatoes may be left to ripen in a fruit bowl and then stored in the refrigerator once they are ripe.

No matter where you live, it is best to buy locally grown seasonal vegetables, which usually have more flavour and cost less than those grown out of season or brought in from far away. Remember to develop a friendly relationship with your greengrocer. You can really help each other.

Frozen and canned vegetables are an appropriate substitute for fresh ones if you feel that the quality of the fresh vegetables available to you is poor or if occasionally time is really short. Manufacturers of both frozen and canned vegetables do their best to preserve the maximum quality and nutritive value of the vegetables they process. However, I believe these foods to be a second choice since their taste is usually affected during the processing. The quality of some canned vegetables such as tomatoes, beans and chick peas is quite acceptable in many dishes.

Simple ways of preparing vegetables

Most of us, especially those cooking for children, prepare vegetables in simple ways, by microwaving, steaming or boiling. The wok is a particularly useful aid to busy people, and you will soon get accustomed to cooking vegetables in it. Many people also enjoy golden brown roast vegetables, and I can tell you how to get great results using a minimum of oil.

Microwaving, steaming and boiling

Microwaving and steaming are excellent techniques because they serve to retain most of the goodness of the vegetables, as long as the vegetables are not overcooked. Those wishing to learn about microwaving will obviously benefit from attending a special class on the subject, where they will receive information on which utensils to use, cooking times, and how to get the most out of the microwave oven.

A large steamer is a timesaver in any kitchen, as you can cook several vegetables and even meat in it at the same time, as well as being able to easily remove some of the food from the steamer without disturbing the cooking of the other ingredients. To cook vegetables

Fresh mushrooms do not need peeling. Just wash them briefly in water.

Make the most of your microwave. Join a microwave cooking class if necessary.

in a steamer, pour some liquid (water, stock or broth) into the lower compartment of the steamer and bring the liquid to the boil. Place the vegetables in the steaming compartment, cover the steamer, and cook until the vegetables are just tender. Some vegetables take longer than others, so occasionally you need to check the level of the steaming liquid.

Alternatively, you can quite efficiently 'steam-cook' vegetables in a small quantity of liquid in a covered saucepan. For instance, bring to the boil 2 or 3 tbsp of water in a saucepan, add some washed broccoli, cover the saucepan, and cook until the broccoli is tender. This technique is particularly suited to cooking spinach. Use a gentle heat and keep your eye on it to prevent your vegetables burning. Boiling vegetables in a large amount of water is really only appropriate if both the liquid and vegetables are to be consumed; for example, when preparing a soup. Many of you would know that some of the water-soluble vitamins are released into the cooking liquid, only to be lost if this precious liquid is then poured down the sink.

Wok cooking

Cooking vegetables in a wok is really exciting because the cook gets so involved, and the vegetables have a popular and distinctively fresh flavour. You will be surprised at how quickly you can prepare a wholesome meal for the whole family using a wok. When cooking in a wok you need to cut the vegetables into regular, bite-size pieces. This must be done before you begin to cook, as the process is quick once you start cooking. First, heat the wok. Then pour a minimum amount of oil into the hot wok. I believe that no more than 1–1½ tbsp of oil is necessary for a stir-fry dish for four people. Peanut oil is favoured by Asian people and, luckily, is also smiled upon by nutritionists.

When stir-frying a vegetable mix, start cooking the hard vegetables first. Cook vegetables such as carrot and celery for about 1½ mins before adding softer vegetables, like cauliflower and broccoli. Then add the very soft ones, like bean sprouts, and last of all shredded cabbage. If the vegetables start to brown or burn, add a little water, say 2 or 3 tbsp, pouring it down the inside of the wok. Stir well and finish the cooking by steaming; that is, by covering the wok with a lid for just a few minutes. The vegetables should still have a crispy texture and the green vegetables should be bright.

When you start to stir-fry you can always flavour the oil, if you wish, by adding some crushed garlic or a crushed slice of ginger, some spices such as a few cummin seeds or aniseeds, or a dried chilli. Towards

Cutting your vegetables on a generous-sized chopping board will reduce the job.

Crisp, stir-fried vegetables and instant noodles make a quick Asian-style meal. Sprinkle with fresh chives or coriander for extra flavour.

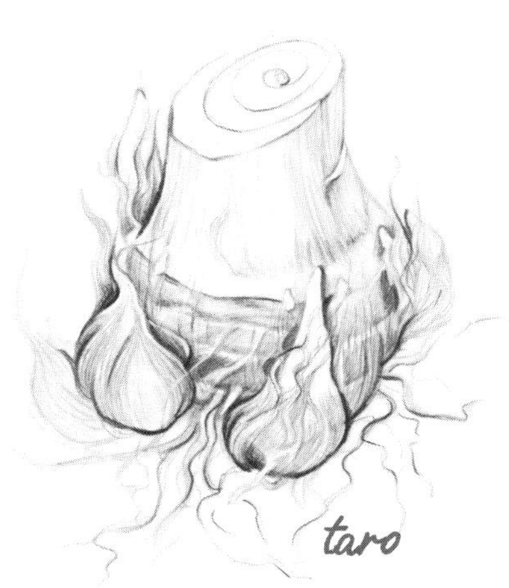

taro

the end of the cooking the vegetables may be seasoned with a little salt-reduced soy sauce and/or some herbs, such as coriander or parsley.

Roasting

How do you roast vegetables? This has to be the question most often asked by my students and it usually comes up during discussions about ways to avoid cooking vegetables in the fat of the meat roast. This is how I roast my vegetables. First, I make sure that I cut my washed, unpeeled vegetables, such as carrots, pumpkin, sweet potatoes, potatoes and taro, into even pieces, and it is easier if the pieces are no larger than an egg. I then toss the vegetables in a tablespoon of olive oil, peanut oil or polyunsaturated oil in a large oven dish, making sure that all sides of the vegetables are lightly coated. I like to season the vegetables with a little paprika and black pepper. Then I place the vegetables on an oven rack set in an oven dish and bake them on the top shelf of my oven while the meat roast cooks on the shelf underneath. The oven is usually set at a moderate temperature of 150°C/ 300°F and the vegetables are roasted and golden brown after about 45 to 50 mins. When roasting vegetables on their own, that is, with no meat cooking at the same time, place them in the centre of the oven set at about 200°C/400°F and the vegetables will cook a little more quickly.

French beans à la provençale

My father grew large quantities of beans and at the end of summer we would bring baskets full of them to the local canning factory, where they would be canned for us in readiness for the cold winter ahead. But here we have beans all year round. The term 'à la provençale' means the way it is done in Provence, a beautiful sunny region in the south of France.

SERVES 4

500 g (about 1 lb) fine French beans

1 small clove garlic, chopped

2 tbsp chopped parsley

a small pinch of salt

1 tbsp olive oil

freshly ground black pepper

Wash beans and top and tail them by hand, removing any strings at the same time. Steam or microwave beans until just tender.

Stir garlic, parsley and salt together.

Brush a large frying pan with oil and add drained beans, garlic, parsley and salt. Toss until vegetables are well coated with herbs, and season with a little pepper before serving.

Cauliflower with pistachios

Pistachio nuts are the seeds of the pistachio tree and are pale green, sweet and delicately nutty in flavour. Adding them to cauliflower is an example of the simple, quick touches that can transform a vegetable into a special-occasion dish.

SERVES ABOUT 4

about ½ cauliflower or enough for 4 people

½ cup water

1 tsp cornflour mixed with 1 tbsp water

1 tbsp quark (cheese)

1 tbsp grated low-fat tasty cheese

a large pinch of grated nutmeg

a pinch of cayenne pepper

1 tbsp raw pistachios cut into small pieces

Cut cauliflower into small flowerets and wash in cold water. Place in a saucepan with ½ cup water, cover pan and steam cauliflower until just soft. Leave liquid in saucepan and place cooked cauliflower in a serving dish and keep warm.

Return pan to high heat and reduce the cooking liquid to about 3 to 4 tbsp. Stir in diluted cornflour and boil until it thickens. Stir in cheese, nutmeg and cayenne and pour this smooth sauce over cauliflower. Sprinkle with pistachios and place dish under a hot grill to very lightly brown the nuts. Serve immediately.

Stir-fried asparagus and mushrooms with bean sprouts

Asparagus and mushrooms are a classic vegetable combination. This stylish dish provides a light entrée for a special occasion, as the photograph opposite page 117 illustrates.

SERVES ABOUT 4

16–20 small to medium asparagus spears

150 g (5 oz) mushrooms (preferably oyster mushrooms)

about 100 g (3½ oz) bean sprouts

¼ red capsicum

1 tbsp peanut or polyunsaturated oil

1 thin slice ginger

1 clove garlic

2 tbsp water

1 tsp salt-reduced soy sauce

Peel larger asparagus spears (small ones need no trimming), starting from just under the head and descending to the base. Regardless of their size, you need to snap off the tough part at the base of the stem. Cut asparagus diagonally into 5 cm (2 in) slices and halve thick pieces lengthwise.

Steam asparagus for 1 min.

Wash mushrooms.

Wash bean sprouts and discard any blemished ones.

Wash and cut capsicum into small squares.

Heat a wok for a few seconds, then add oil and heat it. Add slice of ginger and clove of garlic, asparagus and capsicum, and stir-fry for about 30 secs. Add mushrooms and stir-fry on high heat for 1 min. Add bean sprouts, stir well, add water, cover and cook until asparagus spears are tender.

Remove ginger and garlic and stir in soy sauce just before serving.

Carrot ragoût with gremolata

Gremolata is an Italian seasoning made of parsley, lemon rind and garlic. It is often used to season the traditional osso buco. This stew is simple and inexpensive to prepare.

SERVES ABOUT 4

4 medium carrots

½ brown onion

1 small stick celery

1 tomato

1 tsp olive oil

1 tsp plain flour

1 cup veal or chicken stock (chapter 7) or water

freshly ground black pepper

grated rind of ½ lemon

2 tbsp chopped parsley

1 clove garlic, chopped

Peel and slice carrots (young clean carrots can be used unpeeled).

Peel and chop onion.

Wash and chop celery.

Wash and dice tomato.

Brush a saucepan with oil and gently fry onion and celery for about 2 mins. Stir in flour and tomato, then add carrot and stock. Bring to boil, cover and cook until carrot is tender. Stir in a little pepper, lemon rind, parsley and garlic and serve.

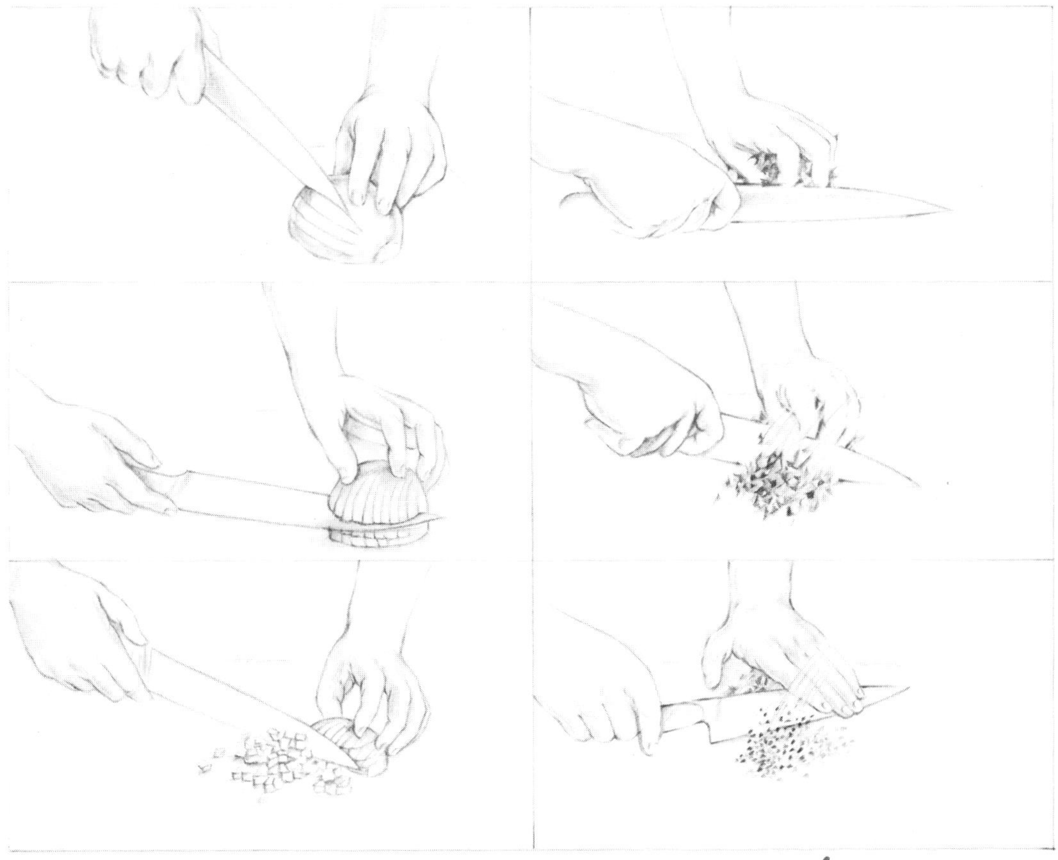

onion

parsley

Stir-fried snow peas with pepitas

Snow peas are ideal if time is short. They literally only take 1 or 2 mins to cook – if cooked longer they lose their delicate flavour and colour. Pepitas (husked pumpkin seeds) are available from supermarkets, nut shops and health-food stores.

SERVES ABOUT 4

400 g (14 oz) snow peas
1 tbsp peanut or polyunsaturated oil
½ clove garlic, crushed
¼ cup water or chicken stock (chapter 7)
a few drops sesame oil
2 tbsp pepitas

Wash snow peas and top and tail by hand.

Heat wok for a few seconds, then heat oil in wok. When hot, add garlic and snow peas and stir-fry for about 1 min. As the snow peas are very delicate, take care not to scorch them. Add water down the inside of the wok, cover and cook on high heat for 1 or 2 mins until snow peas are just tender.

Gently mix in sesame oil and pepitas and serve.

SERVING SUGGESTION: Serve with grilled meat.

Stir-fried broccoli and capsicum with sesame seeds

This beautiful dish of contrasts is popular with lovers of vegetables.

SERVES ABOUT 4

400 g (14 oz) broccoli
1 red capsicum
1 tbsp peanut oil
1 small clove garlic, crushed
1 thin slice ginger
½ cup water
1 tsp salt-reduced soy sauce
a few drops sesame oil
1 tbsp sesame seeds

Wash broccoli, divide into flowerets and then into bite-size pieces by cutting the stalks diagonally.

Halve, seed and wash capsicum and cut into bite-size squares.

Heat oil in hot wok and when oil is hot, add garlic, ginger and broccoli and stir-fry for 1 min. Add capsicum and stir-fry for another minute before adding water. Cover and cook for 2 to 3 mins or until broccoli is tender. Stir in soy sauce, sesame oil and sesame seeds and remove ginger before serving.

Parisian baked tomatoes

Parisian cuisine is one that has been borrowed from all the different regions of France as well as from other countries of the world. The traditional Parisian baked tomatoes contain sausage meat, truffles and mushrooms. In Australia I use minced pork, madeira wine and mushrooms and the dish provides a light, quick meal.

SERVES 1

4 mushrooms

1 tbsp water

2 medium tomatoes

100 g (3½ oz) lean minced pork

1 tbsp madeira wine (optional)

2 tbsp wholemeal breadcrumbs

1 tbsp chopped parsley

freshly ground black pepper

Wash and finely dice mushrooms. Place in a small saucepan with 1 tbsp water and cook for 2 mins. Allow to cool in the liquid.

Preheat oven to 180°C/350°F.

Wash tomatoes and slice off the tops. Scoop out the flesh and reserve it for another use.

In a bowl thoroughly mix pork, diced mushrooms with their juice, madeira, breadcrumbs, parsley and a little pepper. Spoon this stuffing into tomato shells. Place in an oven dish and bake for about 20 mins or until meat is cooked.

Indian-style tomatoes and spinach

If you are familiar with my cookbooks you have probably realised that I love spinach. This is another easy way to prepare it, if you need an imaginative dish in a hurry.

SERVES ABOUT 4

1 bunch spinach

½ brown onion

2 cloves garlic

4 medium tomatoes

1 tsp peanut oil

1 tsp finely grated ginger

¼ tsp fennel seeds

¼ tsp ground cummin

¼ tsp ground turmeric

½ tsp ground coriander

1 tbsp sultanas

¼ tsp hot chilli paste

Detach spinach leaves from stalks and wash leaves two or three times in a large quantity of cold water, then drain.

Peel and chop onion and garlic.

Wash and halve tomatoes and squeeze out the seeds. Chop tomatoes finely.

Brush a large saucepan with oil and on low heat cook onion, garlic and ginger for about 2 mins. Stir in fennel seeds, cummin, turmeric and coriander and cook for 2 mins before adding tomato and sultanas. Bring to boil and cook for 5 mins before adding spinach. Cook, stirring occasionally, until spinach has softened. Season with chilli paste and serve with bread.

Mushrooms and vegetables with herbs

This is a lovely mix of fresh vegetables with just a hint of herbs, easily put together and sure to become a family favourite. We enjoy it served from the centre of the table with roast beef, grilled meats or fish.

SERVES 4

1 medium carrot

½ brown onion

1 stick celery

a few sprigs parsley

a few basil leaves or a few tarragon leaves

1 clove garlic

400 g (14 oz) mushrooms

a handful of spinach or silver beet

a little olive oil

freshly ground black pepper

Peel and finely dice carrot, onion and celery.

Wash and chop parsley, and finely slice basil.

Peel and chop garlic.

Wash and slice mushrooms, leaving very small ones whole.

Wash and finely slice spinach.

Brush a wide saucepan with a little olive oil and, while stirring continuously on medium heat, cook carrot, onion and celery until they soften a little. Increase heat, add mushrooms and cook for a few minutes, stirring occasionally. Add spinach and cook until soft. Stir in parsley, basil and garlic, and season with a little pepper.

Country omelette

This is a very quick, economical meal especially if you use leftover cooked vegetables, such as spinach, beans and broccoli. You can adapt this recipe according to what you have in your refrigerator. Although eggs are a convenient source of protein, remember that it is recommended to moderate our average consumption of eggs to three or four per person per week. Using a black omelette pan or a non-stick pan usually gives the best results.

SERVES 1

1 egg

1 tbsp low-fat milk

3 mushrooms

1 small zucchini

1 tomato

¼ onion

1 tsp peanut oil

freshly ground black pepper

1 tbsp chopped parsley or basil

In a mixing bowl beat egg and milk with a fork until mixture is runny.

Peel and finely slice mushrooms.

Wash and dice zucchini.

Wash, trim and dice tomato.

Peel and finely slice onion.

Brush pan with oil and cook onion for 2 mins, stirring with a wooden spoon. Add mushroom, zucchini and tomato and cook until soft. This only takes a few minutes. Season with a little pepper, and add parsley. Add beaten egg and milk mixture and finish cooking on high heat, stirring well to allow the egg to cook quickly. When all the egg is set the omelette is ready.

SERVING SUGGESTION: Serve with wholegrain bread and a green salad.

▷

Crunchy vegetables, a simple dressing and a scattering of cashew nuts for a swift salad with great style (page 44)

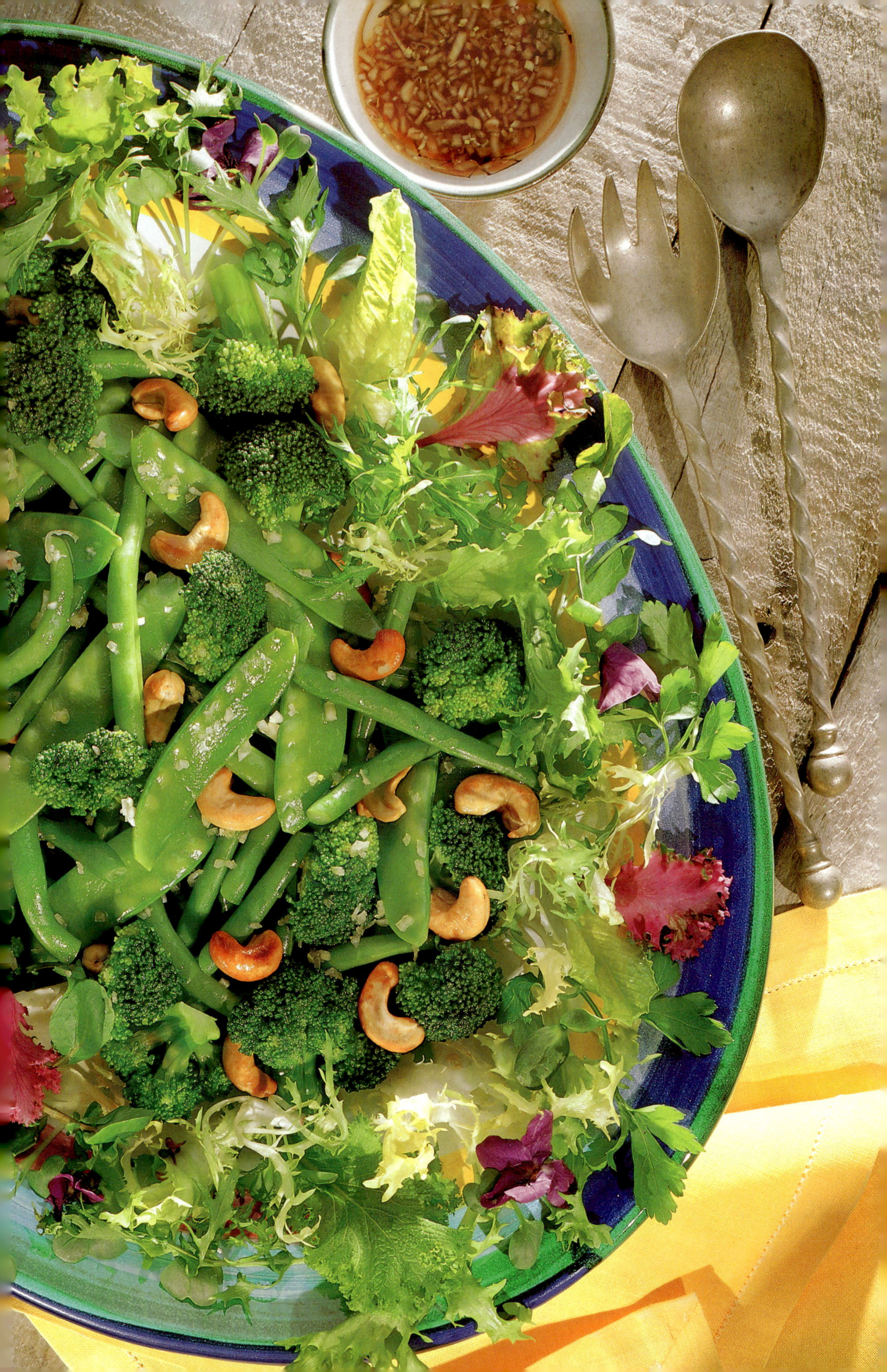

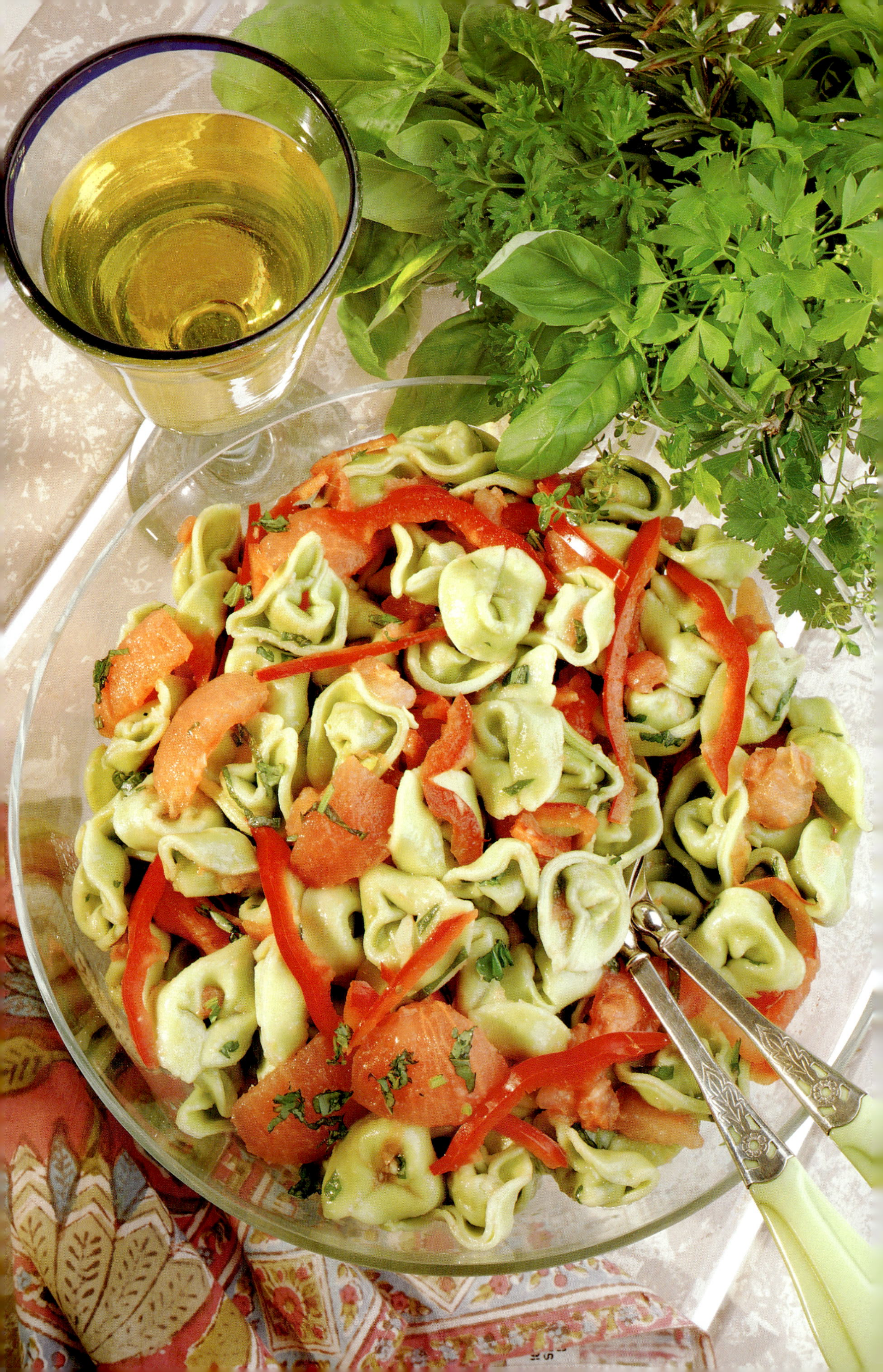

Barbecued vegetables

Barbecued vegetables are always very popular and a light, delicious, easy-to-prepare addition to our traditional barbecued meats. The vegetables are best seasoned a little in advance so perhaps you should prepare them before lighting the barbecue.

SERVES ABOUT 4

2 zucchini

2 small eggplants

4 large mushrooms

1 tsp lemon thyme

2 tbsp polyunsaturated oil

freshly ground black pepper

Wash all vegetables.

Halve zucchini and eggplants lengthwise. Score the cut surface of the vegetable halves with a criss-cross pattern.

Cut off and discard mushroom stalks.

In a large bowl mix lemon thyme, oil and a little pepper and gently toss vegetables with this seasoning. Place vegetables on a clean hot barbecue and cook on both sides until they soften and can be easily pierced with the blade of a knife.

SERVING SUGGESTION: Serve with meat kebabs and rice salad.

Vegetable kebabs

Variety is the spice of life! Vegetable kebabs are great and, served with meat kebabs, make for a balanced barbecue menu. Enlist some help and it will take only minutes to thread them. Remember to soak some bamboo sticks in water for at least 30 mins before using them to prevent burning.

MAKES ABOUT 8
KEBABS

1 clove garlic

6 basil leaves

1 tbsp olive oil

¼ tsp hot chilli paste (optional)

1 green capsicum

1 small brown onion

16 cherry tomatoes

16 mushrooms, about 2 cm (¾ in) in diameter

Peel and finely chop garlic.

Chop basil finely. In a medium bowl mix together garlic, basil, oil and chilli.

Halve, seed and wash capsicum and cut into squares about the same size as the mushrooms.

Peel and halve onion and cut into squares about the same size as the capsicum and mushrooms.

Wash tomatoes and mushrooms.

Toss all vegetables with the flavoured oil then thread vegetables onto sticks, starting with a mushroom and alternating the rest of the vegetables as you go. Refrigerate if not using immediately.

Place kebabs on a very clean, hot barbecue or under the grill and cook for about 4 mins on each side.

◁

A perfect, fuss-free summer lunch — tortellini and red pepper salad, scattered with fresh herbs (page 48)

Mediterranean fennel

This Mediterranean-style dish can be adapted to your family's taste by using your favourite spices and herbs.

SERVES ABOUT 4

2 globes fennel

2 carrots

½ brown onion

¼ tsp cummin seeds (optional)

1 tsp olive oil

1 tsp plain flour

freshly ground black pepper

2 cups beef or chicken stock (chapter 7) or water

2 tbsp chopped parsley

2 tomatoes, sliced

Trim fennel of any damaged leaves and of green ends. Wash and quarter fennel.

Peel and dice carrots and onion.

Place carrot, onion, cummin seeds and oil in a medium saucepan and, using a wooden spoon, gently stir on low heat for 3 mins. Add flour, stir well, then place fennel on top of vegetables. Season with a little pepper and add stock. Sprinkle with parsley, top with sliced tomato, cover and simmer for about 30 mins or until fennel is tender.

SERVING SUGGESTION: Serve with grilled loin of lamb.

Leeks à la grecque

Leeks are usually better in the colder months, and you should always try to choose small ones with very green tops. Braising is a cooking method in which food is cooked in a covered pan with a small amount of liquid.

SERVES ABOUT 4

2–4 leeks

150 g (5 oz) button mushrooms

2 tomatoes

2 tsp olive oil

10 cummin seeds

juice of 1 lemon

¼ cup water

½ tsp dried oregano

Remove damaged or stringy outer leaves of leeks and trim off most of the tougher green parts and the hairy roots at the base. Cut leeks in four lengthwise, leaving the base intact and wash thoroughly in lukewarm water to remove the grit. Cut leeks into 5 cm (2 in) pieces.

Wash mushrooms and slice tomatoes.

Brush a saucepan with olive oil. Sprinkle cummin seeds into dish then add leeks, mushrooms, tomato slices, lemon juice and water. Lastly, sprinkle in oregano.

Bring to boil, reduce to a simmer, cover and cook until leeks are tender. This takes about 15 mins.

Spicy eggplant casserole

At certain times of the year you may find long, thin eggplants at your fruit market. These are a different variety from the rounder eggplants and are usually less bitter.

SERVES ABOUT 4

3 tomatoes

8 long, thin eggplants

½ brown onion

1 clove garlic

1 tsp oil

½ tsp fennel seeds

2 tsp curry powder

4 tbsp wholemeal breadcrumbs

1 tbsp fresh coriander leaves or 1 tbsp flat-leaved parsley

Wash and core tomatoes and blend to a purée.

Trim and wash eggplants. Make a few shallow cuts about 0.6 cm (¼ in) deep in the eggplants.

Peel and chop onion and garlic.

Brush a wide frying pan with oil and gently fry onion, garlic and fennel seeds for 2 mins. Stir in curry powder and cook for about 30 secs before adding tomato purée. Stir well and add breadcrumbs and eggplants. Shake pan well, cover and cook for about 20 mins, turning eggplants over a couple of times during cooking. Cook until eggplants are tender.

Serve sprinkled with coriander leaves.

Sweet and spicy American vegetable casserole

Whether from the north or the south, all the vegetables used in this hearty casserole are native to the Americas. A can of corn is a quick substitute for a cob.

SERVES ABOUT 4

1 red capsicum

1 cob of corn

2 tomatoes

2 medium sweet potatoes (preferably the orange variety)

a little olive oil

about 8 cummin seeds

½ cup water

a pinch of saffron

1 tsp hot chilli paste (optional)

1 tbsp fresh coriander leaves or 1 tbsp flat-leaved parsley (optional)

Halve, seed, wash and finely slice capsicum.

Using a small knife, remove corn kernels from cob.

Wash tomatoes, trim cores and dice tomatoes.

Peel, wash and slice sweet potatoes.

Brush a saucepan with olive oil and on medium heat gently fry capsicum and cummin seeds for 2 mins. Add corn kernels, tomato, sweet potato and ½ cup water. Bring to boil, stir in saffron, cover pan and cook until potato is soft. This takes about 10 mins.

If you wish, stir in chilli paste and coriander leaves before serving.

The humble spud

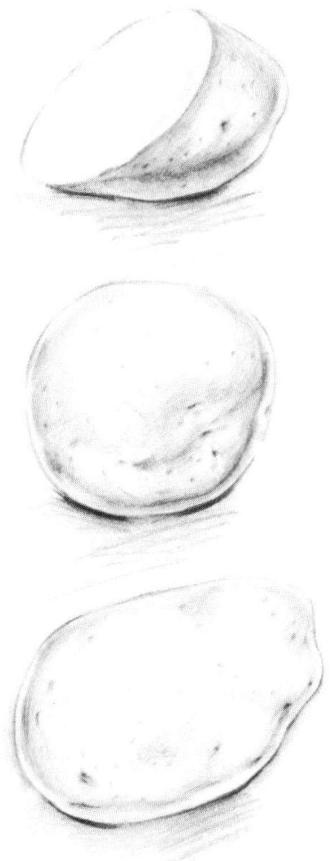

Potatoes are an excellent food for all. They are particularly favoured by athletes, as the starch they contain is digested and absorbed quite slowly and this is beneficial in maintaining a steadier blood sugar level. When cooked in their jackets and not overcooked, potatoes are also a good source of vitamin C. Steaming, microwaving, boiling and baking potatoes in their jackets are the healthiest ways to cook them. Regularly eating deepfried potatoes is something to be avoided, as much fat is absorbed by the potatoes during the cooking.

A great deal of research is currently under way to develop different varieties of potatoes that can be used in varying ways in the kitchen, and greengrocers are slowly introducing a wider choice. Some shopkeepers do need a little encouragement from their customers in this regard, so if we all begin to ask for the new varieties now available, the situation can only improve. Greengrocers themselves can help by labelling potatoes with their real names; for example, 'Pontiac' instead of 'red potatoes'. The types of potatoes available to you depend in some measure on where you live, and the following list of commonly available potatoes describes their main characteristics. I obtained most of the information about potatoes from the Potato Research Station near Healesville, Victoria, where Toolangi Delight and Coliban were bred.

SEBAGO: First bred in the United States, the Sebago is a good all-round potato and popular in home cooking. It is oval in shape and has a white, creamy skin with white flesh.

DESIREE: First developed in the Netherlands, the Desiree potato has a long oval shape with a smooth red-orange skin and pale-yellow flesh. It has good cooking qualities and is excellent for roasting and in potato salad. Avoid overcooking.

SEQUOIA: First bred in the United States, the Sequoia potato has a white flesh with a smooth, creamy yellow skin and a thick, short, oval shape. It is commonly sold as the 'new' potato and is recommended for boiling or for use in salads.

PONTIAC: First introduced in the United States, the Pontiac produces a good yield of regular, round tubers with red skin and white flesh. It makes good potato salad.

KENNEBEC: First developed in the United States, this popular, long, evenly shaped potato has smooth, white skin and white flesh. It is an excellent table potato that has been the principal variety used in making crisps and French fries.

TOOLANGI DELIGHT: This is a popular potato for home growers and cooks alike. The Toolangi has a mostly round shape, a deep-purple skin and white flesh and is suitable for salads, and for mashing, boiling and roasting. What a ripper!

COLIBAN: This potato has a round shape with bright-white skin and white flesh. Its good texture and flavour show little discoloration after cooking, and it is easy to mash and bake.

Warm Toolangi Delight potato salad

Toolangi Delight is a deep purple, mostly round variety of potato. This salad can be enjoyed warm or cold.

SERVES ABOUT 4

3 Toolangi Delight potatoes
about 12 French beans
1 cup cauliflower pieces
1 carrot
1 tsp red wine vinegar
freshly ground black pepper
1 shallot or ¼ white onion, chopped
1 tbsp olive oil
3 tbsp chervil leaves

Wash potatoes and place them in a saucepan, cover with cold water, and cook on medium heat.

Top and tail beans.

Cut cauliflower into small flowerets.

Peel carrot.

Steam beans, cauliflower and carrot.

Peel warm potatoes and cut into cubes. Cut beans and carrots into bite-size pieces.

In a salad bowl mix vinegar, a little pepper, shallot and olive oil and toss vegetables in dressing. Gently stir in chervil leaves and serve.

Curried potatoes with peas and tomatoes

Eaten with bread, this dish can provide a quick, light dinner if you have had an ample lunch. You can replace the peas with another vegetable such as diced carrot, celery or small pieces of cauliflower. If time is really precious you could use frozen peas.

SERVES 4

1 small onion
1 clove garlic
3 tomatoes
4 medium potatoes
1 tsp peanut oil
¼ tsp cummin seeds
2 tsp curry powder
about 1½ cups shelled peas
2 tbsp chopped parsley

Peel and finely chop onion and garlic.

Wash and core tomatoes. Blend to a purée or chop finely. Peel and dice potatoes.

Heat oil in a saucepan and cook onion and garlic on medium heat for a few minutes until onion becomes transparent. Add cummin seeds and stir well for about 10 secs before stirring in curry powder and potato. Add tomato and peas, stir well, cover and simmer gently for about 10 mins or until potato is soft. If using frozen peas, add them 3 to 4 mins before the end. Stir occasionally to make sure mixture doesn't stick to base of saucepan.

Stir in chopped parsley and serve.

Baked potatoes with a creamy topping

The creamy topping is made using quark, a delicious low-fat fresh soft cheese that can be flavoured with herbs or spices of your choice. For instance, for an Italian flavour, try oregano and for a Hungarian touch, use paprika. You need to plan ahead. Put the potatoes in the oven to cook for 40 to 50 mins while you prepare the rest of the meal. The creamy topping only takes a moment to add, just before serving.

SERVES 4

4 large potatoes

1 tbsp low-fat natural yoghurt

3 tbsp quark (fresh low-fat soft cheese with a milk-fat content of less than 8 per cent)

1 tbsp low-fat milk

freshly ground black pepper

a pinch of cayenne pepper

1 tsp grated lemon rind

Preheat oven to 200°C/400°F.

Wash potatoes, place on an oven rack and bake in oven until soft. This takes 40 to 50 mins. Alternatively, you can wrap potatoes in foil and bake in oven.

Blend or whip yoghurt, soft cheese and milk, and season with pepper, cayenne and lemon rind.

Cut a cross about 1 cm (⅓ in) deep in the top of each potato and squeeze the potatoes slightly to make a small opening. Spoon a little topping into this opening and serve.

Sweet potato and avocado purée

This is a nourishing sweet vegetable dish that is best when blended to a very smooth consistency. The addition of herbs gives it a touch of class.

SERVES ABOUT 4

about 500 g (about 1 lb) sweet potatoes (preferably the orange variety)

½ cup water

½ avocado

¼ tsp curry powder

2 tbsp chopped parsley

freshly ground black pepper

Peel and cut sweet potatoes into bite-size pieces. Place in a saucepan with the water, cover and cook until potato is soft.

Remove sweet potato from liquid and blend with peeled avocado and curry powder to a very smooth purée. If it is too dry, add a little cooking liquid from the sweet potato. Stir in parsley, season with a little black pepper and serve.

SERVING SUGGESTION: Serve with a roast accompanied by green vegetables and bread.

Salad Days

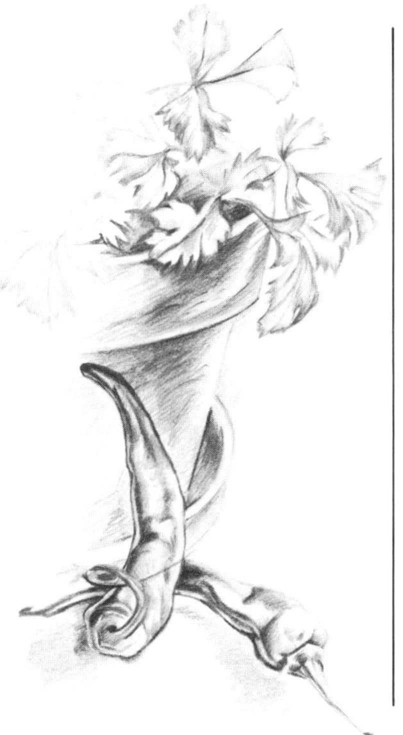

Being a keen vegetable gardener for the past forty years, my father has always provided the family table with a variety of seasonal vegetables. Among other things, he grows the most tender beans, the sweetest tomatoes and some very appetising greens that my mother transforms into a daily salad, whether it be a scorching hot day or a day on which the roof of the house is blanketed under a few centimetres of snow.

I still have vivid memories of the way we went about preparing the salad. *Maman* would wash the greens and one or more of the children would help by drying the salad in the salad spinner, fetching the herbs from the garden, or mixing and tasting the salad dressing. I remember loving the aroma of red wine vinegar and the dedicated way my grandmother used to gently toss the salad once it was ready. Nowadays, my children somehow seem to enjoy the same little jobs that I did.

Making a quick meal with a salad

There is, of course, the salad sandwich, made with wholemeal or wholegrain bread, so satisfying and easy to prepare and providing good energy. But you can also mix a more substantial salad without much last-minute effort if you are prepared to plan a little in advance. For example, are you going to cook pasta, potatoes, rice or pulses for tonight's dinner? Well, if so, cook a little extra and keep it for a salad for tomorrow. These foods will provide the bulk of your dish, and you just need to add a few leafy greens, some raw vegetables, grated or sliced, and some cold meat or fish. Such a combination provides a lovely contrast of texture and flavour and with a tangy dressing of spices and herbs makes an exciting meal.

Crunchy oriental salad with cashews

For a pleasant green vegetable salad, the vegetables must be just cooked and still crunchy. This salad is very popular for barbecues. I usually serve it from a large platter decorated with a few leafy greens, as in our photograph opposite page 36.

SERVES ABOUT 4

about 200 g (7 oz) snow peas

about 200 g (7 oz) French beans

about 200 g (7 oz) broccoli

1 tsp red wine vinegar

¼ white onion, finely chopped

freshly ground black pepper

1 tbsp cashew nuts

1 tbsp peanut or polyunsaturated oil

½ tsp sesame oil

Wash and top and tail snow peas and beans.

Wash broccoli and cut into bite-size pieces.

Separately steam, boil or microwave the three vegetables until just cooked. The snow peas take the least amount of time to cook and the beans take the longest. Place vegetables in ice-cold water for long enough to cool them. Drain vegetables and then dry them a little using a clean teatowel.

In a salad bowl mix vinegar, onion, a little pepper, cashews and oils. Gently toss vegetables in dressing just before serving.

Apollo Bay summer salad

This salad is dedicated to an organic vegetable grower from Apollo Bay who delights us every summer with outstanding sweet tomatoes with tender, thin skins. We regularly prepare this quick salad for lunch on warm days.

SERVES ABOUT 4

200 g (7 oz) French beans

a few leafy greens

4 medium tomatoes

2 medium potatoes, cooked

1 tsp red wine vinegar

freshly ground black pepper

1 tbsp olive oil

about 6 basil leaves, finely sliced

String, wash and cook beans, either by steaming, microwaving or boiling them. Place cooked beans in cold water and then drain.

Wash and dry leafy greens.

Wash tomatoes, trim eyes and quarter tomatoes.

Peel and slice potatoes.

In a salad bowl mix vinegar, a little pepper and olive oil. Add beans, greens, tomato and potato. Toss well and serve sprinkled with basil.

Aussie luncheon salad

Many of us consume an unnecessarily large quantity of meat. If we are going to have meat, chicken or fish for dinner, it is nutritionally adequate to eat a meatless lunch, say a salad sandwich or, at home, a mixed salad accompanied by good bread. This salad makes a lovely light lunch for those days when you are on the run.

SERVES 4

juice of 1 lemon
freshly ground black pepper
1 tbsp peanut oil
a few cos lettuce leaves or
other greens
2 medium carrots
2 tomatoes
1 avocado
2 tbsp walnuts

In a salad bowl mix lemon juice, a little pepper and oil.

Wash lettuce and dry leaves well. Tear leaves into 2 or 3 pieces and place in the salad bowl.

Peel and finely grate carrots and add to bowl.

Trim and dice tomatoes and add to bowl.

Halve avocado and remove stone. Peel and dice avocado and add to bowl. Add walnuts and toss salad gently just before serving.

Witlof, walnut and egg salad

Witlof has a very attractive, refreshing bitterness. It is important to choose witlof with yellow-tipped leaves. If green, they are not good.

SERVES ABOUT 4

4 small witlof
2 hard-boiled eggs
1 tsp red wine vinegar
2 pinches of curry powder
1 shallot or ¼ white onion,
finely chopped
1 tbsp peanut or
polyunsaturated oil
2 tbsp chopped walnuts
1 tbsp chopped parsley

Wash and finely slice witlof.

Peel eggs and slice thinly. Use an egg cutter if you have one.

In a salad bowl, mix red wine vinegar, curry powder and shallot and then mix in oil.

Gently toss witlof with egg, chopped walnuts and dressing, sprinkle with parsley and serve.

Red cabbage, spinach and carrot salad

This is an anti-cancer salad par excellence. Cabbage, carrots and spinach are good sources of fibre and their vitamins are believed to help protect the body from cancer. For this salad choose small spinach leaves that are young and tender.

SERVES 4–6

about 20 small spinach leaves

½ fresh red cabbage

1 medium carrot

1 tbsp red wine vinegar

freshly ground black pepper

**1 tbsp peanut or
polyunsaturated oil**

1 tbsp sultanas

Wash spinach two or three times in a large quantity of cold water. Drain and dry spinach leaves in a teatowel or salad spinner.

Trim core of cabbage and remove any damaged leaves. Wash and finely shred cabbage using a large knife or a food processor.

Peel and grate carrot.

In a large bowl, mix vinegar, a little pepper and oil. Add spinach leaves, cabbage, carrot and sultanas and toss gently before serving.

Thai cabbage and bean sprout salad

I owe the inspiration for this quick salad to our friends Shirley and Frank, who once served a similar dish at a wonderful Asian dinner.

SERVES ABOUT 4

¼ Chinese cabbage

a handful bean sprouts

**a 10 cm (4 in) stalk lemon
grass, finely chopped**

juice of 2 limes or 1 lemon

1 tbsp Asian fish sauce

**1 red chilli pepper, halved,
seeded and finely sliced**

1 clove garlic, chopped

1 tsp peanut oil

**2 tbsp fresh coriander leaves
or 2 tbsp flat-leaved parsley**

Bring a large saucepan of water to the boil.

Trim thick stalk of cabbage, then wash and finely shred cabbage. Cook for 2 mins in boiling water, then drain and refresh cabbage by rinsing in cold water for a few minutes. Drain again.

Wash bean sprouts and remove any damaged ones.

In a large bowl combine lemon grass, lime juice, fish sauce, chilli, garlic and oil. Toss drained cabbage and bean shoots in the dressing and sprinkle with coriander leaves.

Japanese radish salad with ginger

The long white Japanese variety of radish, resembling a long turnip, is available in oriental food stores and also at many greengrocers. To shred the radish, I use the shredding attachment of my food processor, which saves time, but you can also use a knife or grater.

SERVES ABOUT 4

1 Japanese radish

1 small carrot

juice of ½ lemon

a 2 cm (¾ in) piece of ginger

¼ tsp sesame oil

1 tbsp peanut oil

1 tsp salt-reduced soy sauce

freshly ground black pepper

Peel and shred radish and carrot and mix well with lemon juice.

Peel, slice and cut ginger into fine strips.

In a salad bowl, mix sesame oil, peanut oil, soy sauce, ginger and a little pepper. Toss radish and carrot in dressing.

Creamy carrot and walnut dip

This is an ideal light start to a special-occasion meal when the main dish is fairly robust. The soft cheese used in this dip is low in fat and made from skim milk and a culture. It is the Australian version of the German quark or the French fromage blanc, and the varieties available in supermarkets and delis here have a milk-fat content of less than 8 per cent. With this dip serve a selection of pieces of raw vegetables, such as celery, radish, carrot, cauliflower, capsicum, zucchini, and witlof leaves, or serve it with good bread.

SERVES ABOUT 8

1 medium carrot

2 tbsp walnut meat

4 tbsp quark (fresh low-fat soft cheese with a milk-fat content of less than 8 per cent)

1 tbsp low-fat milk

¼ tsp curry powder

a few drops lemon juice

freshly ground black pepper

Peel and finely grate carrot.

Place walnuts in a food processor and blend briefly so walnuts are in small pieces. Add cheese, milk, curry powder, carrot, lemon juice and a little pepper and blend until ingredients are well combined.

If you don't have a food processor beat cheese with milk, curry powder, lemon juice and pepper until smooth, then add finely chopped walnuts and grated carrot and mix well together.

Serve with your selection of raw vegetables.

Tortellini and red pepper salad

Tortellini is an Italian pasta filled with meat. For a lovely effect, use green spinach-flavoured tortellini and red capsicum. If fresh or dried tortellini is unavailable you can substitute frozen varieties. This salad is simple to prepare yet substantial enough to serve as a main course, as the photograph opposite page 37 demonstrates.

SERVES ABOUT 4

1 red capsicum

2 tomatoes

1 tsp balsamic vinegar

1 tbsp olive oil

1 clove garlic, chopped

freshly ground black pepper

250 g (9 oz) fresh green tortellini

6 basil leaves, finely sliced

Halve, seed and wash capsicum and slice very finely.

Wash and cut tomatoes into small pieces.

In a salad bowl mix capsicum and tomato with vinegar, oil, garlic and a little pepper.

Bring a large saucepan of lightly salted water to the boil and cook tortellini until tender (it takes 8 to 12 mins, depending on the dryness of the pasta) or cook according to packet instructions.

Drain cooked tortellini and cool in very cold water. Drain again and gently shake to remove as much water as possible. Then gently stir tortellini into salad bowl with finely sliced basil, and serve.

Curried aromatic rice salad

I enjoy this salad with cold meat. You can be creative with the flavour of your curry by varying the spices here or by using spices of your own choice. Cook the rice the day before required or at least a few hours beforehand to allow it to cool.

SERVES ABOUT 4

1–1½ tbsp peanut oil

1 brown onion, finely chopped

¼ tsp cummin seeds

1 tsp curry powder

½ tsp turmeric

1 cup basmati rice

1¾ cups cold water

1 apple

1 banana

juice of 1 lemon

2 tbsp fresh coriander leaves or 2 tbsp flat-leaved parsley

Brush a medium saucepan with ½ tbsp oil and when oil is hot gently fry onion and cummin seeds for 2 mins. Add curry powder and turmeric and stir for 1 min. Add rice, stir and add 1¾ cups cold water. Bring to a simmer, cover and cook on low heat for about 17 mins or until rice is tender. Check water level once or twice during cooking and add a little hot water if necessary.

Allow rice to cool.

Wash, quarter, core and slice apple. Peel and slice banana.

In a salad bowl mix lemon juice and remaining peanut oil. Add rice and separate the grains using a spoon. Gently toss with apple and banana and sprinkle with coriander leaves.

Pontiac potato and corn salad

Pontiac potatoes are ideal for salads and they rarely darken after cooking. If you are in a hurry and make this salad just before the meal, serve it lukewarm – it tastes even better. A can of corn is an acceptable substitute for fresh corn at busy times.

SERVES ABOUT 4

4 medium Pontiac potatoes
1 cob of corn
1 shallot or ½ white onion
1 tbsp vinegar
freshly ground black pepper
1 tbsp olive oil
1 tbsp snipped chives
1 tbsp chopped parsley

Wash and steam, boil or microwave potatoes in their skins until just cooked.

Steam, boil or microwave corn. If boiling it, you may cook it in the same water as the potatoes. The corn cooks in 5 to 8 mins.

Peel and chop shallot.

Using a small knife, remove corn kernels from cob.

In a salad bowl, mix together vinegar, shallots, a little pepper and oil.

Peel and halve potatoes and cut into slices. Gently toss with dressing, corn, chives and parsley.

Moroccan chick peas with coriander

The easiest and quickest way to prepare this salad is to use canned (cooked) chick peas. But if you have time to plan, it is not difficult to cook your own chick peas.

SERVES ABOUT 4

1 cup dried chick peas or about 2 cups cooked chick peas
½ cup fresh coriander leaves
1 tbsp pine nuts
1 tbsp low-fat natural yoghurt
1 tbsp low-fat milk
¼ tsp hot chilli paste or a pinch of chilli powder
½ red capsicum (optional)
2 spring onions

If using uncooked chick peas, soak them overnight then discard the soaking water and cook chick peas in four times their volume of water. It takes 2 to 3 hrs, unless you have a pressure cooker, in which case it can be done in 45 mins to 1 hr. The peas look better and have a more agreeable texture if they are cooked slowly. Allow them to cool in the cooking liquid, then drain them.

In a small food processor blend coriander leaves, pine nuts, yoghurt, milk and chilli paste to a purée. Alternatively, chop coriander leaves and pine nuts finely and mix well with yoghurt, milk and chilli paste.

Wash capsicum, remove seeds and slice capsicum finely.

Wash spring onions and cut into small pieces.

In a salad bowl gently toss chick peas, capsicum and spring onion with the coriander dressing.

Soupe du Jour

We have often heartened friends (and ourselves) with the simplest of vegetable soups, such as the carrot soup that is in this chapter. For the cook, a soup is an easy entrée for a special-occasion meal and is always a versatile choice, for almost any dish can follow a light soup.

For most home cooks a soup is often planned as a meal in itself, since this saves time in food preparation. So we open our fridge. What have we got? As if for a puzzle, we begin to assemble a few pieces of vegetables: there may be a zucchini, a carrot, a piece of cabbage and a leek, and with the help of a few potatoes or a can of cooked beans or chick peas, or perhaps some cooked rice or small pasta, we quickly create something delicious. Served with wholesome bread, such a meal makes us feel really good.

Soups should be an important part of the repertoire of a busy cook. Soup can be a meal, so there is no need to prepare other courses, and most soups heat up brilliantly in minutes for a meal the next day.

Soup can make the perfect one-dish meal.

Modifying soup recipes

If you are following a soup recipe from a book, read the instructions carefully to establish whether you will need to modify the dish to make it suitable for the occasion you have in mind. If the soup is to be the first of several courses, the amount of fat used should be kept to a minimum. For instance, in a creamed asparagus or pumpkin or broccoli soup, you can replace the 2 tbsp of cream or butter, which is traditionally added at the end, by 1 tbsp of powdered skim milk diluted with 1 tbsp of water or milk. Try also to reduce the amount of salt added to the soup. If the preparation includes bacon or another type of salted meat, or cheese, added salt is simply unnecessary. However, if you must add salt, do so at

Keep chicken stock in the freezer as a base for quick, flavoursome soups.

the beginning of the recipe. A small pinch of salt added early in the cooking is more effective than several pinches at the end, as it helps release the flavour of the ingredients into the liquid. Before serving, I season my soups with a little black pepper or another spice, or with finely sliced or chopped herbs. I favour parsley and chives with smooth soups but prefer basil and coriander in more chunky soups.

If your soup is intended as a meal, consider whether it will provide a good balance of ingredients that will be nutritious enough. If necessary, you can modify a dish by introducing new ingredients. To a mixed vegetable soup the addition of a can of cooked beans, lentils or chick peas is delightful, and especially nutritious when served with wholegrain bread. A little grated cheese is also most welcome. At home I use cold roast chicken or pork and cooked rice or small pasta in soups to create some lovely concoctions.

French provincial soup

Once you are a little experienced in everyday soupmaking, you don't need to follow a recipe but can simply use whatever vegetables you have on hand in the refrigerator. Remember that potatoes always make a good soup ingredient. And be relaxed. Try out new vegetables, experiment, and enjoy your cooking.

SERVES ABOUT 4

1 carrot

1 turnip

1 stick celery

a handful French beans

2 medium potatoes

1 tsp olive or peanut oil

4–8 fennel seeds

2 tbsp chopped parsley

1 small clove garlic, finely chopped (optional)

freshly ground black pepper

Peel and dice carrot and turnip.

Wash and dice celery and beans.

Peel, wash and dice potatoes.

Heat oil in a saucepan and gently fry carrot, celery and fennel seeds for 3 to 4 mins. Add turnip and potato, cover with water and bring to boil. Add beans and cook for about 15 mins until potato is tender.

Add chopped parsley and garlic, season with a little pepper and serve.

Thai prawn and noodle soup

This quick, tasty soup can be partly prepared in advance, leaving the cook with very little last-minute preparation. You'll see a photograph of the soup opposite page 4.

SERVES 4

8–12 green prawns

a little peanut oil

6 cups water

1 stalk finely sliced lemon grass or 1 tbsp grated lemon rind

1 carrot, finely sliced

60 g (2 oz) cellophane noodles

juice of 1 lemon or 1 lime

1 tbsp Asian fish sauce

1–3 fresh chillies, seeded and finely sliced

2 tbsp fresh coriander leaves or 2 tbsp flat-leaved parsley

4 spring onions, cut into 2.5 cm (1 in) pieces

Shell and devein prawns.

Brush a large saucepan with oil. Add prawn shells, including heads, and stir for about 3 mins on high heat. Add water and lemon grass, bring to boil and cook for a further 10 mins. Strain, discarding prawn shells, and return liquid to pan. Bring to boil, add carrot and cook for 1 min before adding noodles. Stir gently and add prawns, lemon juice, fish sauce and chilli. Allow prawns to cook for about 2 mins without allowing the liquid to boil.

Stir in coriander leaves and spring onions just before serving.

Carrot soup

For a balance of sweetness and flavour use medium-sized carrots for this simple but classic soup. Transform the soup into a meal by adding a can of cooked chick peas. Just reheat the soup and eat it with good bread. If you would like the soup to be a little creamier, stir in 1 tbsp of powdered skim milk mixed with 1 tbsp of cold water just before serving.

SERVES ABOUT 4

1 small brown onion

about 6 medium carrots

a little polyunsaturated oil

4 cups chicken stock (chapter 7) or water

a small pinch of salt

freshly ground black pepper

2 tbsp chopped parsley or chives

▷

Entertaining with ease – honeyed oriental drumsticks (page 102) and a refreshing, chilled watercress soup (page 55)

Peel and dice onion.

Peel carrots and cut into small pieces.

Brush a large saucepan with a little oil and gently fry onion for a few minutes. Add cold stock or water, salt and carrot. Bring to boil, cover and cook until carrot is soft. It takes about 15 mins.

Blend soup to a fine purée. Reheat soup, season with a little black pepper and stir in parsley or chives before serving.

SERVING SUGGESTION: Serve with wholemeal or wholegrain bread.

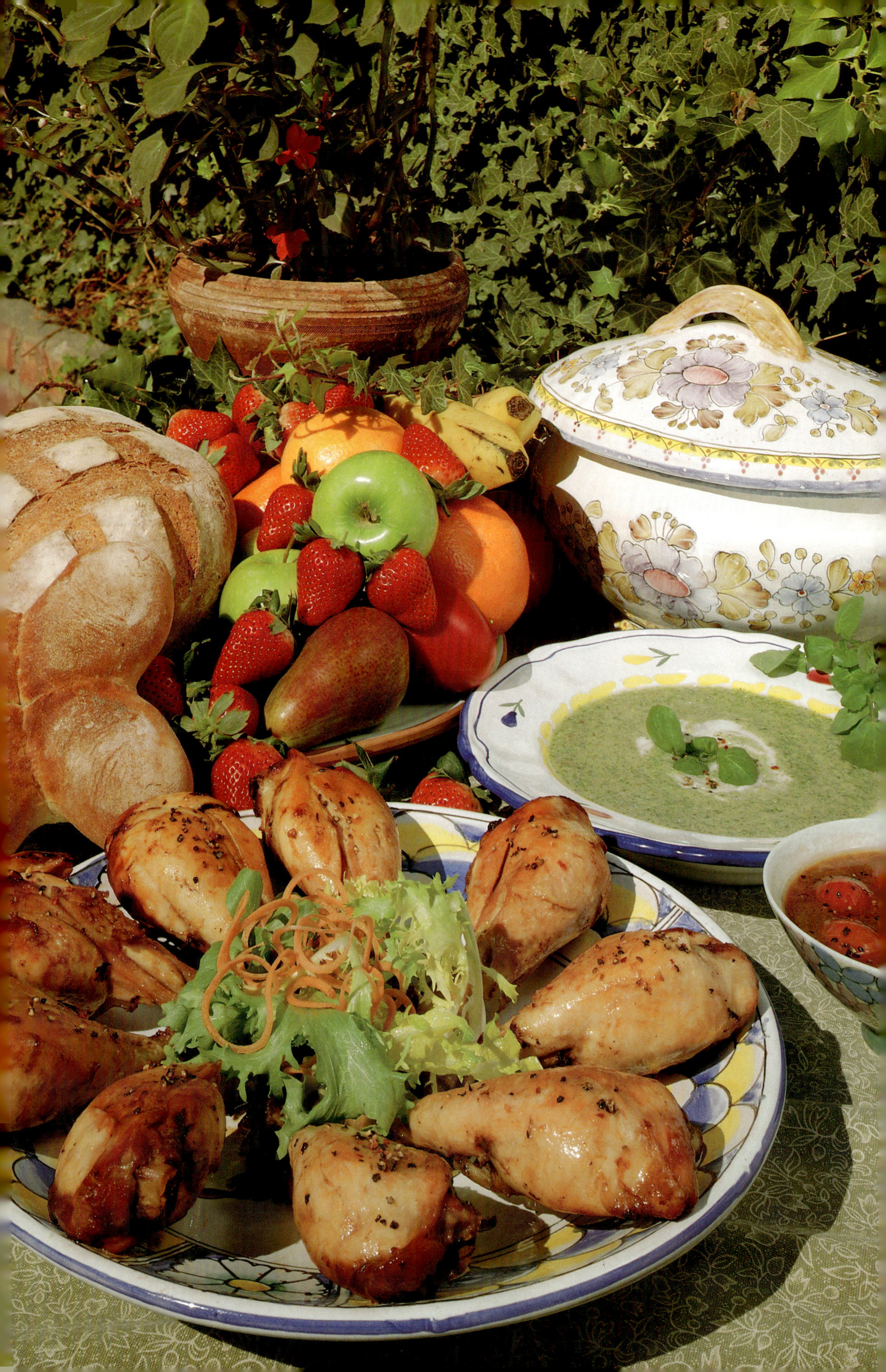

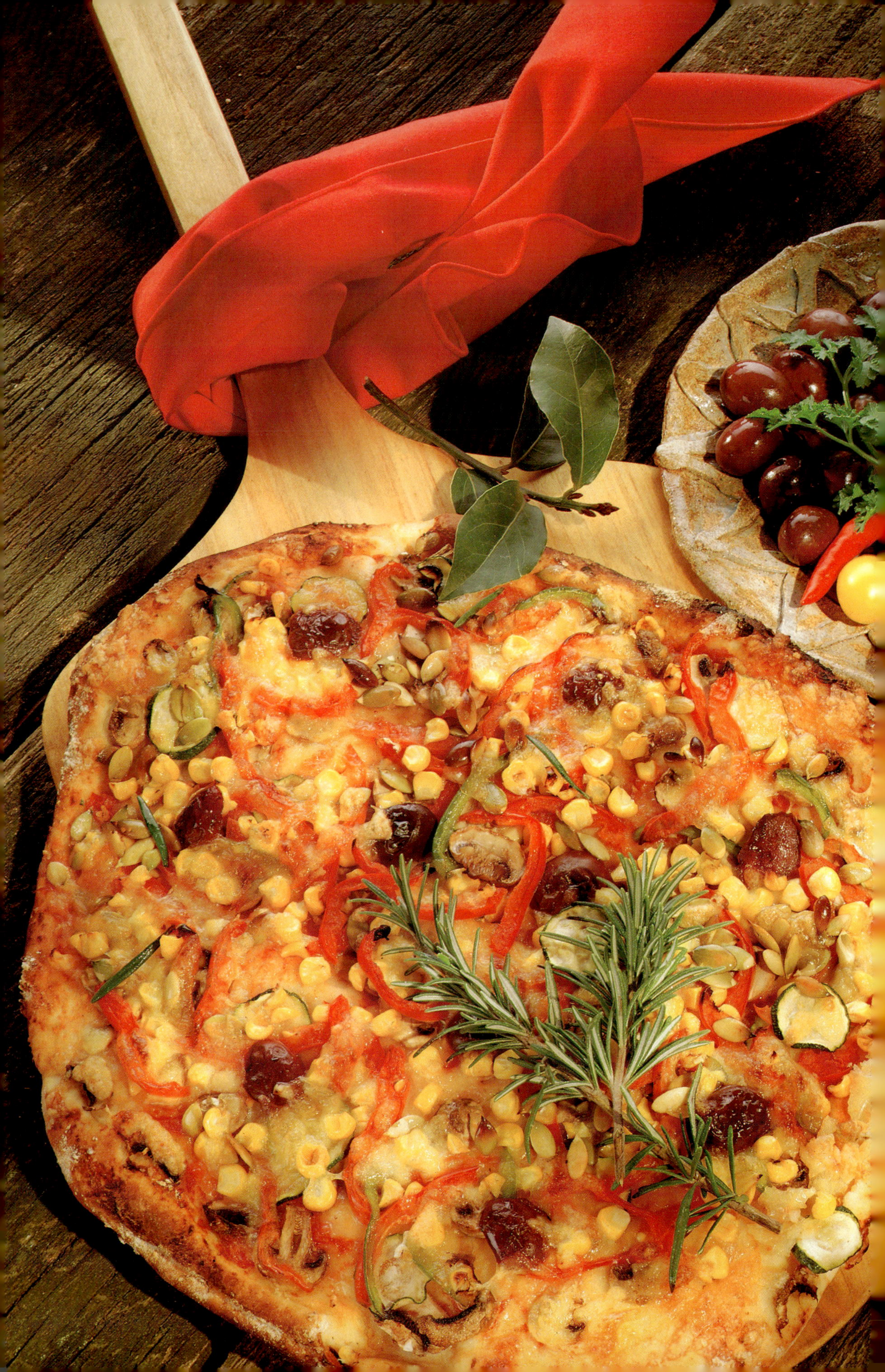

French green pea and lettuce soup

Green pea soup with lettuce is a French classic and is always eaten with bread. It requires a minimum of time to make yet it has the most marvellous flavour. In my version I have included a little pumpkin and carrot to obtain the smoothness and sweetness traditionally achieved by adding cream.

SERVES ABOUT 4

1 medium carrot

about 1 cup pumpkin flesh

1 small brown onion

1 butter lettuce or ¼ larger lettuce

1 tsp peanut oil

a pinch of salt

a pinch of curry powder

4 cups chicken stock (chapter 7)

1½ cups shelled peas (or frozen peas)

2 tbsp chopped parsley

freshly ground black pepper

Peel carrot. Cut pumpkin and carrot into small pieces about the size of peas.

Peel and chop onion.

Wash and finely slice lettuce.

Brush a large saucepan with oil and gently fry onion for a few minutes. Add a pinch of salt, curry powder, carrot, pumpkin and lettuce and stir for 2 mins. Add stock, bring to boil, and boil for 5 mins. Add peas and boil uncovered until peas are soft. This takes 8 to 10 mins.

Blend soup to a smooth purée. Reheat soup, stir in parsley and season with a little black pepper just before serving.

SERVING SUGGESTION: Serve with wholegrain bread.

Scottish vegetable and oat soup

In Scotland oats are a very popular soup ingredient. They are growing in popularity here now, as the type of fibre they contain is reputed to be beneficial in lowering blood cholesterol in addition to its high-fibre properties. This soup is fast but filling.

SERVES ABOUT 4

1 medium leek

1 medium carrot

2 cups pumpkin flesh

½ tsp peanut or polyunsaturated oil

5 cups cold water

a small pinch of salt

1 cup rolled oats

2 tbsp chopped parsley

freshly ground black pepper

Cut leek in four lengthwise, leaving root intact, and wash thoroughly in lukewarm water to remove grit.

Peel carrot and cut in four lengthwise. Cut carrot and leek into small slices.

Cut pumpkin into small pieces.

Heat oil in a large saucepan and on low heat gently fry leek and carrot for about 5 mins, stirring continuously, using a wooden spoon. Add cold water, salt and pumpkin, bring to boil and cook for a further 5 mins. Add rolled oats and boil for another 15 mins. Stir in parsley and season with a little pepper just before serving.

◁

Easy-make, easy-bake pizza, hearty and wholesome, with loads of fresh vegetables (page 78)

Italian vegetable and vermicelli soup

This Italian-style soup is a light meal that I enjoy for lunch in winter served with crusty bread. The addition of cooked chicken or cooked dried beans makes it heartier.

SERVES 4

1 carrot

100 g (3½ oz) French beans

1 zucchini

1 stick celery

1 cup cauliflower pieces

a little olive oil

½ tsp finely chopped rosemary

5 cups water

1 cup vermicelli or other small pasta

6 basil leaves

1 clove garlic

1 tbsp grated parmesan cheese

freshly ground black pepper

Trim and peel carrot.

Top and tail beans.

Trim zucchini.

Wash celery and cauliflower.

Cut carrot, zucchini and celery into slices and cut beans and cauliflower into bite-size pieces.

Brush a saucepan with oil and gently fry rosemary, carrot, zucchini and celery for a few minutes. Add beans, cauliflower and water and boil for 2 mins before adding pasta. Stir well, return to boil and cook for 10 mins.

Finely chop basil and garlic. Stir basil, garlic and parmesan into soup and season with a little pepper just before serving.

Noumean leek and taro soup

My last visit to Nouméa inspired me to prepare this satisfying soup, which is delicious with bread. Taro is available from most greengrocers and Asian grocers. It is a root vegetable not unlike sweet potato. If taro is not available, substitute sweet potatoes or potatoes.

SERVES ABOUT 4

1 medium leek

1 medium carrot

a 400 g (14 oz) taro

1 tsp olive oil

¼ tsp fennel seeds

4 cups cold water

a small pinch of salt

a pinch of cayenne pepper

2 tbsp chopped parsley

1 clove garlic, chopped (optional)

Cut leek in four lengthwise, leaving root intact and wash leek thoroughly in lukewarm water to remove grit.

Peel carrot and halve lengthwise before cutting into small slices.

Peel taro and cut lengthwise into sticks about 1 cm (⅓ in) thick, then into very fine slices.

Heat oil in a large saucepan and on low heat add fennel seeds, leek and carrot and stir gently for a minute or so. Add the cold water, salt and taro and bring to boil. Cook soup for 15 to 20 mins until vegetables are soft.

Just before serving, stir in cayenne pepper, parsley and garlic.

Chinese corn and chilli fish soup

This unusual soup is smooth and delicate, and provides a light meal or, served in small quantities, an elegant first course for a special occasion. Once the fish is added to the soup, reheat without boiling the liquid, otherwise the fish will lose its tenderness. You can save a few minutes by substituting a can of corn for the cobs.

SERVES ABOUT 4

1 medium leek

1 small stick celery

1 medium carrot

about 250 g (9 oz) skinned fish fillet

1 tbsp salt-reduced soy sauce

1 tsp cornflour

a little peanut oil

4 cups chicken stock (chapter 7) or vegetable broth

2 cobs of corn

1 tbsp chopped parsley

¼ tsp hot chilli paste (optional)

freshly ground black pepper

Cut leek in four lengthwise, leaving root intact. Wash leek thoroughly in lukewarm water to remove grit. Remove any damaged outer leaves and slice leek thinly.

Wash and dice celery.

Peel carrot and cut in four lengthwise before slicing thinly.

Cut fish into bite-size pieces. Discard any bones.

Brush a saucepan with a little oil and gently fry sliced leek, celery and carrot for 3 to 4 mins. Add stock and bring to boil.

Wash corn and, using a small sharp knife, remove kernels from cob. Add corn to soup and cook until all vegetables are tender.

Blend about one-third of the soup to a fine purée. Return purée to pan and bring soup to a light simmer. Stir in fish pieces, turn off heat, cover pan and leave for 2 mins. Then stir in parsley, chilli paste and a little pepper and serve.

Chilled watercress soup

Watercress has a refreshing peppery flavour and when mixed with cucumber, smooth soft cheese and bread it becomes a delectable light meal. It is perfect for those summery days when you would rather relax with family and friends than be inside cooking. If you are in a great rush, replace the carrot with an extra tomato. This soup is in the photograph opposite page 52.

SERVES 4–8

1 medium carrot

3 tbsp water

4 slices wholemeal bread

1 cup low-fat milk

1 European cucumber, the slim variety

2 cups watercress

1 tomato

2 tbsp quark (cheese)

Peel and dice carrot and place in a small saucepan with the water. Cover and cook until carrot is soft, then allow to cool.

Soak bread in milk.

Peel cucumber and halve it lengthwise. Remove seeds and cut cucumber into 8 pieces.

Wash watercress in cold water and remove any damaged stalks and leaves.

Wash tomato, trim eye and quarter tomato.

Blend to a purée the cold carrot with its liquid, soaked bread and milk, cucumber, watercress, tomato and cheese. If you wish, thin the soup with more milk.

Chilled celery and avocado soup

This is one of the fastest soups I know of. It can be made in a flash, yet it has an irresistible creamy texture and subtle flavour. I like to use celery from the heart of the bunch, as the centre stalks are a little more tender than the outside ones.

SERVES ABOUT 3

2 slices wholemeal bread

1 cup vegetable stock or water

1½ cups celery pieces

1 ripe avocado

juice of ½ lemon

2 tbsp bottled or home-made Italian tomato sauce (chapter 7)

½ cup low-fat natural yoghurt

¼ tsp hot chilli paste

a small pinch of salt

2 tbsp snipped chives

freshly ground black pepper

Cut bread into small pieces and soak in the vegetable stock.

Wash celery.

Peel avocado and cut into pieces.

Blend soaked bread and stock, celery, avocado, lemon juice, tomato sauce, yoghurt, chilli paste and salt to a smooth consistency. If necessary, add a little water to obtain a soup texture.

Chill, stir in chives and a little pepper and serve.

Tangy summer tomato and sweet potato soup

This is a cold soup to commence a summer dinner party or to eat as a light meal with bread. The flavour is sweet and spicy and has the exotic aftertaste of coriander leaves.

SERVES ABOUT 4

1 brown onion

1 small carrot

1 small stick celery

400 g (14 oz) ripe tomatoes

½–1 tbsp peanut or polyunsaturated oil

¼ tsp cummin seeds

3 cups chicken stock (chapter 7) or water

1 orange sweet potato

freshly ground black pepper

¼ tsp hot chilli paste

1 tbsp fresh coriander leaves or 1 tbsp flat-leaved parsley

Peel and dice onion, carrot and celery.

Wash tomatoes and cut them into quarters.

In a medium saucepan heat oil and on low heat sauté onion, carrot, celery and cummin seeds for about 5 mins, stirring occasionally. Add tomato and chicken stock and bring to a gentle boil.

Peel and dice sweet potato, add to boiling soup and cook uncovered for about 15 mins.

Blend soup to a purée or press through a sieve. Cool soup and refrigerate if not using straight away.

Season soup with a little pepper and chilli paste and sprinkle with coriander leaves before serving.

Chunky chicken and vegetable soup

This soup is a one-pot meal and is, therefore, easy to prepare. Use any vegetables you have on hand if you do not have those suggested. The soup appears opposite page 21.

SERVES ABOUT 4

1 small leek

2 medium carrots

1 zucchini

1 stick celery

100 g (3½ oz) broccoli or cauliflower or both

a little olive oil

6 cups water

1 cup pasta (e.g. butterfly, springs)

300 g (11 oz) deboned chicken pieces (fillet or thigh)

1 tbsp chopped parsley

freshly ground black pepper

Cut leek in four lengthwise, leaving the root intact. Wash leek thoroughly in lukewarm water to remove grit. Slice leek thinly.

Peel carrots and slice thinly.

Wash zucchini and celery and slice both thinly.

Wash broccoli and separate flowerets into bite-size pieces.

Brush a saucepan with a little oil and on medium heat gently fry leek, carrot, zucchini and celery for 2 mins. Add water and return to boil. Add pasta, stir well, bring to boil and cook for about 5 mins.

Meanwhile, skin chicken and cut into bite-size pieces.

Add broccoli to soup and boil for 3 mins. Add chicken pieces and stir well. Keep soup hot for 5 mins to allow the small chicken pieces to cook but avoid boiling, as the chicken will become tough.

Season soup with parsley and a little pepper before serving.

Lentil and vegetable soup

Eaten with wholemeal bread, this is a one-dish meal, made easier by using canned lentils. The vegetables can, of course, be varied depending on what you have in your refrigerator.

SERVES ABOUT 4

½ brown onion

2 carrots

about 1 cup pumpkin flesh

2 medium potatoes

3 zucchini or about 200 g (7 oz) French beans

1 tomato

a little peanut or polyunsaturated oil

6 cups water

a 400 g (14 oz) can lentils

2–3 tbsp chopped parsley

1 clove garlic, finely chopped

freshly ground black pepper

Peel and dice onion, carrots, pumpkin and potatoes.

Wash and slice zucchini.

Wash and dice tomato.

Brush a large saucepan with oil and on low heat fry onion, carrot and zucchini for 3 or 4 mins. Stir in tomato and add water, potato and pumpkin. Bring to boil and cook for about 10 mins. Add drained lentils and cook for a further 5 mins. Stir in parsley and garlic and season with a little pepper just before serving.

Faster Pasta, Pulses and Rice

You may have heard that several worldwide studies have shown that people who eat a vegetarian diet have, in general, fewer diet-related diseases, like cancer and heart disease, than those eating a meat-based diet. These findings must, of course, be interpreted carefully. Many groups of people who are traditionally vegetarian follow healthy life-styles in other important respects such as reduced smoking and alcohol consumption. If a vegetarian diet has a more beneficial effect, this may be because it provides a higher intake of fibre and vitamins and can be lower in saturated fat than a diet high in meat. Such studies do not say that meat is bad for us. What we can learn from them is that whichever diet we choose to adopt, it must provide a good balance of nutrients. Some of us need to eat more high-fibre foods, which are also low in fat. In this chapter you will find dishes of pulses, cereals, rice and pasta, some meatless meals and a few bread recipes.

Vegetarian meals

In our search for an appropriate diet for our family, my wife Angie and I have found that eating regular vegetarian meals has been very pleasant. We prepare dishes of pasta with vegetables, sometimes sprinkled with a little grated parmesan. We also love legumes, like dried beans, split peas and chick peas, cooked in many different ways with vegetables, seasoned with spices and herbs, and served with good bread. Over the past two years we have learned to use cereals such as bourghul (cracked wheat), an important staple food throughout the Middle East, and quinoa, a grain native to South America that is cooked in the same way as rice.

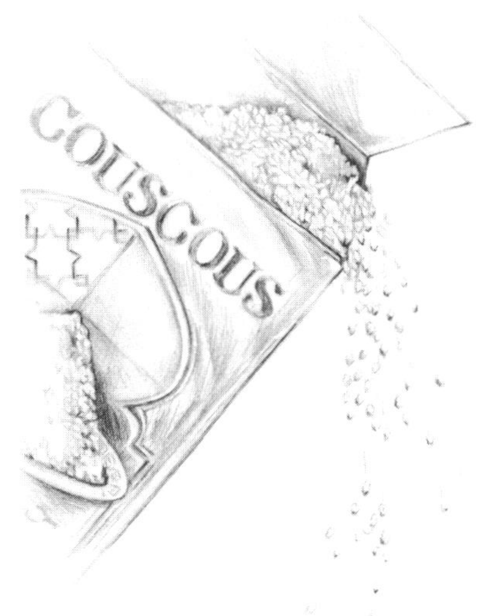

Try strolling through your local supermarket and taking the time to consider the range of pulses and cereals on the shelves. You could probably try a new one every day of the week and you may be surprised to learn that some of them, like lentils, couscous and quinoa, take very little time to cook.

Anyone wanting to change over to a permanent vegetarian diet will definitely benefit from seeking information from the local health department. The guidelines of the Anti–Cancer Council's Prudent Diet apply to vegetarians as well as to non–vegetarians. The most important point is to eat a wide variety of foods in order to obtain all the nutrients we need. Vegetarians, especially vegans, who consume no egg or milk products, must find their protein in a combination of two types of plant foods. Cereal grains (wheat, oats, rice, and so on), nuts and seeds provide one type, while legumes, such as split peas, dried beans and the like, provide the other. You will find many recipes combining these two types of protein in this chapter. Note the importance of bread to accompany dishes based on legumes.

Eggs and dairy products are another excellent source of protein for vegetarians. Vegetarians who do not consume dairy products may experience difficulty in meeting the recommended dietary allowance for calcium, but eating nuts and seeds regularly increases calcium supply.

Meat eaters usually obtain an adequate iron intake but vegetarians need to choose plant sources of this important nutrient. Particularly during pregnancy this may not be sufficient for vegetarian women.

Other sections of this book, for example the vegetable, salad and soup chapters, provide further ideas for preparing vegetarian meals.

Cereals

Cereals are an important food named after Ceres, the Roman goddess of agriculture, and cereal grains of every kind have featured in all traditional diets since the time agriculture began thousands of years ago. The most popular cereal of all is rice, which remains the staple food of half the world's population. The other half relies on wheat, oats, corn and barley, to name a few, which form the basis of hundreds of preparations including bread, pasta, pastries and the like.

In our daily lives there is plenty of opportunity to eat cereal, and in nearly every chapter of this book you will find recipes using one form or another. Flour of course is a common cereal product. Even in the dessert section, rolled oats make for a delicious rhubarb and

Experiment with cereals you have not tried before. Some like quinoa and couscous take only a few minutes to prepare.

blackberry crumble, while corn meal is used to make the orange and polenta custard. However, breakfast seems to be the perfect time of the day to eat cereals. Cereal grains are the usual basis for processed, commercial 'breakfast cereals'; for example, rolled oats, cornflakes, rice bubbles, wheat biscuits and muesli. If processed simply, without extra ingredients such as oil, chocolate and sugar, they are naturally low in fat, especially when consumed with low-fat milk. Cereals are a good source of complex carbohydrate that provides long-lasting energy. Because of their high-fibre content, cereals are particularly recommended by health authorities.

Pasta

In our household pasta comes to the rescue when we need a hot meal in a hurry. Pasta cooks more quickly than rice and potatoes and is always a hit with the young. In terms of nutrition, pasta, made principally of flour and water, is like bread and, therefore, is an excellent source of fibre and B vitamins. Wholemeal pasta offers more goodness and has a nuttier flavour than pasta made from plain flour. If you are unaccustomed to the coarser texture of wholemeal pasta, start with small pasta like macaroni or elbow-shaped pasta, going on to the larger shapes later.

Dried pasta is an essential in any pantry cupboard. If you are really in a hurry, buy fresh pasta. It cooks even more quickly, usually taking just 2 or 3 mins.

Cooking

Cook pasta in a large quantity of lightly salted boiling water. Once the pasta is immersed in the water, give it a brief stir with a wooden spoon to stop it from sticking together, and remember that during cooking the water must boil at all times. Cooking time varies depending on the type of pasta used. Dried pasta takes a little longer than fresh pasta, and, in general, wholemeal pasta take a bit longer than plain flour pasta. The packet instructions should indicate the cooking time, and if you use fresh pasta the shop where you buy it will give you approximate cooking times. To check if pasta is ready, taste it. It should be soft on the outside and just a little firm in the centre. The Italians call it *al dente*. When you are satisfied that your pasta is *al dente*, immediately drain it in a colander, shaking it well to extract all the water trapped in the pasta. Then, depending on the dish you are preparing, return the pasta to the pan or transfer it to a deep serving dish and mix in your seasoning or sauce.

To save time, dried pasta may be cooked in advance. Once it is done, drain the cooked pasta and stop the cooking by putting it in cold water. Then again drain well and place in a bowl until required. Simply reheat the pasta briefly in boiling water before draining it and mixing in your seasoning. Olive oil is a popular fat for seasoning pasta but should be used in moderation as illustrated in the following recipes.

Fettuccine with vegetables and herbs

The choice of vegetables used here is really a matter of taste and may depend on what you have in your refrigerator. If you do have time to plan, the following suggestions can produce beautiful flavours and colours. Our front cover features this recipe.

SERVES ABOUT 4

1 cup broccoli, cut into small pieces

1 tomato

½ red capsicum

½ brown onion

1 small eggplant

6 mushrooms

1 tbsp olive oil

1 clove garlic, chopped

1 tbsp finely sliced basil

1 tbsp chopped parsley

300–400 g (11–14 oz) fettuccine

1 tbsp pine nuts

2 tbsp grated parmesan cheese

Wash broccoli and steam or microwave it until *al dente*, i.e. just cooked but still firm.

Halve tomato and after squeezing out the seeds by hand, dice the flesh.

Wash capsicum, remove seeds and slice capsicum finely.

Peel and slice onion finely.

Wash eggplant and slice finely.

Wash and slice mushrooms.

In a large wok or frying pan heat oil and stir-fry capsicum, onion, eggplant and mushroom until soft. Add broccoli, tomato, garlic, basil and parsley. Gently stir well for 30 secs, turn off heat and keep warm until pasta is cooked.

Cook fettuccine according to packet instructions. Gently stir drained pasta, vegetables and pine nuts together and serve sprinkled with a little grated parmesan cheese.

Sunday macaroni

This is one of our light, regular Sunday evening dishes and macaroni is a favourite pasta shape with our children. Notice the moderate use of bacon. The dish can be transformed into a meal by mixing in cooked diced vegetables.

SERVES ABOUT 4

3–4 cups wholemeal macaroni

1 slice lean bacon

1 tbsp olive oil

2 tbsp pine nuts

1 clove garlic, finely chopped

1 tbsp chopped parsley

1 tbsp finely sliced basil

freshly ground black pepper

2 tbsp grated parmesan cheese

Cook macaroni in lightly salted boiling water, according to packet instructions.

Meanwhile, trim bacon of fat and dice bacon.

Heat oil in a medium saucepan and fry bacon for 1 min on medium heat. Add pine nuts, browning them a little before adding garlic. Stir and remove from heat.

Drain cooked macaroni and shake a little to extract water trapped inside. Mix macaroni with bacon and pine nuts in saucepan and gently stir in parsley and basil. Season with a little pepper. Before serving sprinkle with grated parmesan.

SERVING SUGGESTION: Serve with a mixed salad or steamed green vegetables.

Seashell pasta with mushroom herb sauce

Seashell pasta, or 'conchiglie rigate' in Italian, is special because the sauce you serve with it goes inside the shells, resulting in a beautiful taste experience.

SERVES ABOUT 4

½ brown onion

250 g (9 oz) small button mushrooms

1 tbsp olive oil

½ clove garlic, finely chopped

4 tbsp bottled or home-made Italian tomato sauce (chapter 7)

1 tbsp finely sliced basil

1 tbsp chopped parsley

freshly ground black pepper

1 tbsp pine nuts

3–4 cups seashell pasta, preferably wholemeal

1 tbsp grated parmesan cheese

Peel and finely chop onion.

Wash mushrooms and slice finely.

Heat oil in a frying pan and on high heat fry onion for 1 min. Add mushroom and garlic and, stirring occasionally, cook until mushroom is soft. Add tomato sauce, stir well and boil for 1 min before stirring in basil, parsley, a little pepper and pine nuts.

Cook pasta in lightly salted boiling water, according to packet instructions.

Drain hot pasta and shake gently to extract water trapped inside the pasta shells. Gently mix pasta with hot sauce before serving, and sprinkle with grated parmesan.

Butterfly pasta with chive sauce

It is interesting to compare the differences in flavour of the many varied shapes of pasta now available. Butterfly pasta shapes are soft and slippery with a sauce.

SERVES ABOUT 4

2 tomatoes

300–400 g (11–14 oz) butterfly pasta

1 tbsp olive oil

1 clove garlic, chopped

freshly ground black pepper

2 tbsp grated parmesan cheese

3 tbsp snipped chives

Halve tomatoes and, after squeezing out the seeds by hand, dice the flesh.

Bring a large pot of lightly salted water to the boil and cook pasta in boiling water until *al dente*. Drain pasta when cooked.

Meanwhile, heat olive oil in a saucepan and gently fry garlic for 10 secs. Add tomato and stir-fry for about 2 mins. Stir drained pasta into tomato and season with pepper. Mix in parmesan and chives and serve.

Spaghetti with mushrooms and asparagus

This dish is ideal for a light lunch shared with good friends, especially when you have little time for preparation.

SERVES ABOUT 4

300–400 g (11–14 oz) spaghetti, preferably wholemeal

about 16 small asparagus spears

200 g (7 oz) mushrooms

½ tbsp olive oil

1 small clove garlic, chopped

freshly ground black pepper

2 tbsp chopped parsley

1 tbsp grated parmesan cheese

Bring a large pot of lightly salted water to the boil. Add pasta and cook in boiling water until *al dente*. When cooked, drain pasta.

Meanwhile, wash asparagus and snap off the hard part at the base of each spear. Steam or microwave asparagus until just slightly crunchy.

Wash and slice mushrooms.

Heat olive oil in a large saucepan. With pan on high heat stir in garlic and mushroom and cook until mushroom is soft. It takes 3 to 4 mins. Gently stir in spaghetti and asparagus, season with a little pepper and add parsley.

Serve sprinkled with a little grated parmesan.

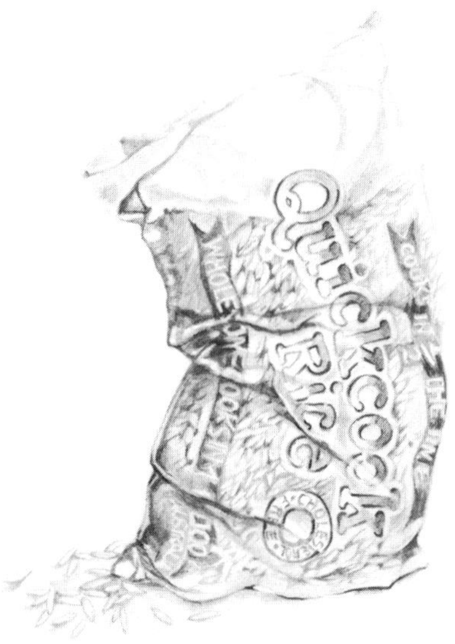

Rice in the kitchen

Rice is a convenient product as it can be stored for a long time without deteriorating. A second advantage is that most children love it. Many of my students have surprised me by saying that they cook rice only if preparing Asian-style dishes. Rice is so versatile! It may be served with many different kinds of foods: it is delicious with poached or grilled fish, with poached chicken, any sauced dishes, with pulses, with vegetables and, of course, in soups and salads. You can even use it to make desserts, as many good, old-fashioned cooks know.

On our pantry shelves at home we always have a selection of rice. In fact, there are hundreds of varieties but they fit into two basic groups: long grain and short grain. Long-grain rice, which tends to be dry and separates after being cooked, is popular in salads and with curries and stews. Short-grain rice is favoured by those who eat using chopsticks because it is moister and the grains stick together, making it easier to pick up. At home we enjoy different varieties of rice and often prepare brown rice, which has a nutty flavour and offers extra nutrition because of its additional fibre and B vitamins. When it comes to white rice, we prefer the long-grain basmati rice whose unique, aromatic flavour we love.

Cooking rice

I prefer to cook rice using the absorption method. Simply place the rice in a saucepan and, if preparing white rice, add one-and-a-half times as much cold water as rice and 1 tsp of polyunsaturated oil. For brown rice, add twice its volume of cold water and 1 tsp of oil. Bring to the boil, lower to a simmer, cover the pan and cook until the rice is tender. Check the level of the water regularly towards the end of the cooking and add a little boiling water from the kettle if necessary. White rice takes about 17 mins to cook. Long-grain brown rice needs about 35 mins, which is a little less time than is required for short-grain brown rice, whose fatter grains require 45 to 50 mins.

Rice can also be boiled in a large volume of lightly salted water, and cooking times are roughly the same as indicated above, but it is wise to read the packet instructions carefully.

Cook extra rice for tomorrow's soup, salad or stuffed vegetables.

Mexican chilli rice with peas

This dish was inspired by a traditional Mexican rice dish called 'anoz verde' ('green rice'), which is deliciously flavoured with herbs, hot chilli and green vegetables. I use brown rice as it is more nutritious.

SERVES ABOUT 4

1 small brown onion, chopped

1 stick celery

½ small green chilli, seeds removed

1 tbsp olive oil

1 cup long-grain brown rice

a pinch of salt

2½ cups chicken stock (chapter 7) or water

about 1 cup shelled peas

3 tbsp chopped parsley

1 tbsp finely sliced fresh coriander leaves or 1 tbsp flat-leaved parsley

Peel and dice onion and celery.

Slice chilli finely.

Heat oil in a large saucepan and on low heat gently fry onion, celery and chilli for about 3 mins. Add rice and stir for 10 secs before adding stock and salt. Bring to boil, reduce to a simmer, cover pan and cook for 20 mins.

After 20 mins has elapsed, gently stir in peas, parsley and coriander. Cover pan and cook for a further 20 mins or until rice is tender.

Basmati rice with spicy apple and walnuts

Here is one of those dishes that was thrown together one day when there was not much left in the fridge. Luckily, I found some basmati rice, some spices and nuts in the pantry and an apple in the fruit bowl. The result was a great success. If you keep your pantry stocked with essentials, you will always be able to prepare a wholesome meal at short notice.

SERVES ABOUT 2

½ cup basmati rice

about 10 caraway seeds

a pinch of salt

2 tbsp sultanas

1¼ cups water

1 apple

2 tbsp walnut meat

½ tbsp peanut or polyunsaturated oil

½ brown onion, chopped

2 tsp curry powder

Place rice, caraway seeds, salt, half the sultanas and water in a small saucepan. Bring to boil, cover and simmer for about 17 mins or until rice is tender.

Meanwhile, peel and dice apple.

Cut walnuts into small pieces.

Heat oil in a small saucepan and gently fry onion for about 2 mins. Add curry powder, stir well for a couple of minutes, then add diced apple and remaining sultanas. Stir again, cover and cook for 3 mins more. Stir in walnut pieces, cook for 1 min then remove from heat.

When rice is cooked, serve it topped with the apple and walnut sauce.

Baked capsicum with rice and tuna

This dish makes a popular light meal for adults and can be quickly prepared, especially if you use cooked rice left over from the previous day. Use canned tuna in oil and drain the oil, or if you prefer a less oily flavour use tuna canned in water.

SERVES 4

4 red or green capsicums

½ brown onion

1 stick celery

½ tbsp olive oil or tuna oil from the can

2 cups cooked rice (preferably brown rice)

2 tbsp chopped parsley

freshly ground black pepper

a 185 g (about 5½ oz) can tuna

Preheat oven to 200°C/400°F.

Open capsicums by cutting off a slice from the longest edge of each. Chop these four slices quite finely. Discard seeds and wash capsicums under tap. Place capsicums in a roasting dish just large enough to hold them and roast in preheated oven for 20 mins.

Peel and chop onion.

Wash and dice celery.

Brush a saucepan with olive oil. Add chopped capsicum, onion and celery and cook on medium heat for about 5 mins, until vegetables are almost soft. Add rice and chopped parsley and season with a little pepper. Stir on low heat for 2 mins then remove from heat and stir in drained tuna, broken into small pieces.

Pack this preparation fairly tightly into the capsicums and bake for a further 10 mins. By that time, the rice and tuna should be hot and the capsicum soft.

Middle Eastern rice with carrots

This delicious vegetarian dish uses only one saucepan and can be adapted to the seasons using vegetables of your choice.

SERVES ABOUT 4

a little olive oil

¼ tsp cummin seeds

1 tomato, finely chopped

1 cup long-grain brown rice

4 cups water

½ cup red lentils

12 small carrots, peeled

1 cup shelled peas

freshly ground black pepper

2 tbsp chopped parsley

Brush a large saucepan with oil. Place pan on low heat, add cummin seeds and cook for 1 min. Add tomato, rice and water, bring to boil, cover pan and cook for 20 mins. Add lentils, cover again and cook for a further 10 mins. Add carrots and peas and again cook for 10 mins. If there is too much liquid left towards the end, remove lid for the last 5 mins of the cooking time.

Season with a little pepper and sprinkle with parsley before serving.

Dried pulses

Although many Australians love baked beans on toast, dried pulses – lentils, dried beans, chick peas – are less popular in Australia than in many other countries, like England, Italy, France, Mexico and the Middle East. This is a pity, for pulses are a convenient and nutritious family food. At our place there are always some packets of dried beans or lentils in the pantry, and a few cans of chick peas and cooked beans for those days when there just doesn't seem to be enough time. Furthermore, pulses are inexpensive and very easy to prepare.

The flexibility that these foods offer is a joy to the cook. Cooked beans can be transformed into a dip, a soup, a salad or a vegetable dish, and they may be embellished with hundreds of different seasonings, like cummin, curry spices, parsley, garlic, and so on. In addition, pulses are often interchangeable in a recipe, so if you do not have the one indicated you can replace it with another.

Cooking pulses

As mentioned earlier, cooking pulses is simple but I know that busy people are sometimes deterred by the fact that most pulses need to be soaked overnight and also require an hour or more to cook, depending on the type, dryness and size of the pulse in question. However, a little planning can help enormously. A reminder written in the diary ('soak beans') may be all that is required, and then the pulses for the following day's meal can be cooked while you are preparing the dinner that evening; or perhaps the weekend might be a good time to do it. Of course, the last resort is to open a can.

With the exception of lentils, all pulses need to be soaked. The traditional method is to soak the pulses for at least 8 to 10 hrs. Note that soy beans need to be soaked for 24 hrs. If time doesn't allow you to soak the pulses in the traditional way, you can place them in unsalted water, bring them to the boil and simmer for 5 mins. Leave them in the water for 1 to 2 hrs, then drain and rinse, and the pulses are ready to be cooked. Lentils and split peas take 20 to 45 mins to cook in three times their volume of water, while most dried beans take about 1 hr in four times their volume of water. Broad beans, chick peas and soy beans take the longest time of all – 2 to 3½ hrs in four times their volume of water.

Sprinkle fresh herbs on pulses for extra flavour: there are lots to choose from.

Canned beans and lentils are a great standby if you don't have time to soak any pulses. Look for the low-salt varieties.

Spicy borlotti and cannellini bean casserole

This easy-to-prepare vegetarian dried bean dish calls for a little planning, as the beans need to soak overnight or for at least 12 hrs. Borlotti beans are reddish with spots while cannellini beans are a creamy white colour. Both varieties are commonly available from supermarkets, health-food stores and continental grocery shops. Other beans can be used or, if you are short of time, use canned beans.

SERVES ABOUT 4–6

½ cup dried borlotti beans or a 400 g (14 oz) can borlotti beans (no added salt), drained

½ cup cannellini beans or a 400 g (14 oz) can cannellini beans (no added salt), drained

1 medium carrot

1 small capsicum (green, red or yellow)

3 tomatoes

½ tbsp peanut oil

½ brown onion, chopped

1 small clove garlic, chopped

1 tsp curry powder

4 cups water

½ cup shelled peas

¼ tsp hot chilli paste (optional)

2 tbsp chopped parsley

Soak borlotti and cannellini beans in a large quantity of cold water for at least 12 hrs.

Peel and slice carrot.

Halve capsicum and discard seeds. Wash and dice capsicum.

Wash, trim and dice tomatoes.

In a saucepan heat oil and gently fry onion and garlic for 2 mins. Add curry powder and stir well before adding carrot, capsicum and tomato. Stir and cook for 1 min before adding water and drained beans. Bring to boil, reduce to a simmer and cook for 50 mins.

Add peas and cook for another 10 mins or so or until beans are tender. Stir in chilli paste and chopped parsley and enjoy with good bread.

Dhal

You might have already tried this lentil purée in an Indian restaurant. Indian families cook their own versions, using various combinations of lentils, herbs, spices and vegetables. My version of this aromatic blend is delicious by itself or as an accompaniment to rice or vegetables. If you wish to save about 15 mins of cooking time, use red lentils only. Despite the long list of ingredients, dhal is simple to prepare, as all the ingredients are tossed into the pot to cook together. You can be doing other things while the dhal simmers for an hour. Dhal accompanies the chicken curry opposite page 100.

SERVES ABOUT 4

a handful spinach

about 1 cup pumpkin pieces

½ cup red lentils

½ cup brown lentils

1 crushed clove or a pinch of ground cloves

1 curry leaf

½ tsp ground cummin

½ tsp ground coriander

a 2 cm (¾ in) stick cinnamon

½ tsp turmeric

1 tsp aniseed

½ brown onion, chopped

1 clove garlic

1 tsp grated ginger

4 cups water

about 20 fresh coriander leaves, finely sliced

1 tbsp finely sliced dill

1 tbsp chopped mint

Wash spinach two or three times in a large quantity of cold water.

Place all ingredients except the coriander, dill and mint into a large saucepan. Bring to a simmer, cover pan and cook until lentils are quite soft. It may take 50 mins to 1 hr.

Remove cinnamon stick and curry leaf. Blend lentils to a purée but not too fine. Reheat in a saucepan and just before serving, stir in coriander, dill and mint.

SERVING SUGGESTION: Serve with rice and Indian breads.

Spanish bourghul and bean stew

Bourghul is the name given to wheat that is cooked and parched before being ground. This nutty grain is very popular in Mediterranean and Middle Eastern cooking and is also the grain used in the traditional tabouli. Don't be daunted by the longish list of ingredients – you will be surprised at how quick this is to make. To save time I have used canned cannellini beans but of course you can cook your own if you prefer.

SERVES ABOUT 4

2 tomatoes or half a 400 g (14 oz) can peeled tomatoes (no added salt), drained

1 small green capsicum

1 tbsp olive oil

1 small brown onion, chopped

1 clove garlic, chopped

1 cup bourghul

a pinch of saffron

½ tsp paprika

a pinch of cayenne pepper

freshly ground black pepper

2 cups water

a 400 g (14 oz) can cannellini beans (no added salt), drained

1 tbsp chopped parsley

Wash and dice tomatoes.

Halve capsicum, remove seeds and slice capsicum into bite-size pieces.

Heat oil in a medium saucepan and on medium heat fry onion for 2 mins. Add garlic, capsicum and bourghul and stir for about 3 mins without browning. Add tomato, saffron, paprika, cayenne pepper and a little pepper. Stir well, add water, bring to boil, cover pan and simmer for 10 mins.

Gently stir in drained beans and parsley and simmer, uncovered, for a few minutes to heat the beans. By this time there should be very little liquid left in the pan.

SERVING SUGGESTION: Serve with steamed spinach.

Quinoa with green beans

Quinoa is a small grain about the same size as coarse semolina. It is high in protein and together with corn and potatoes was a staple food of the Inca civilisation. It is a nutty grain and may be cooked in the same way as rice, taking about 10 to 15 mins to cook. Our children like it.

SERVES ABOUT 4

300 g (11 oz) French beans

1 brown onion

1 tsp olive oil

2 cups water

1 cup quinoa

a pinch of salt

a pinch of cayenne pepper (optional)

freshly ground black pepper

Top and tail beans. Wash beans and cut them in half.

Peel onion and slice finely.

Brush a large saucepan with oil and on low heat gently fry onion for about 3 mins. Add beans and stir-fry on medium heat for a minute or so before adding water, quinoa, salt, cayenne pepper and a little freshly ground black pepper. Bring to a gentle boil, cover and cook for 10 to 12 mins.

Well bread

For instant nourishment it is hard to beat bread. It can turn a simple bowl of soup or a plate of vegetables into a meal. Toasted and crunchy it is lovely for breakfast. With summer-ripe tomatoes and a scattering of fresh basil it is a perfect snack. And it is the basis for an endless variety of wholesome sandwiches.

To make your own bread does take some time and practice. However, once you have mastered the art you will find you can make your favourite bread without a recipe and with a minimum of fuss. And once you have the ingredients and equipment out, it is just as easy to make two or three loaves and freeze some for later use or to share with friends.

The bread recipes in this chapter have been specially created to simplify the task and shorten the time of making bread. Both the kneading and rising time are shorter than in traditional recipes, and I have included one really fast bread recipe for you to try.

Home-made bread

I love making bread at home, for just handling the dough establishes a special link between the food and the cook. The following bread recipes have been very carefully put together with Russell, a jolly friend of mine who is a baker. We have simplified the recipes as much as possible in an attempt to make breadmaking a happy experience for the beginner and to encourage readers to make bread more often. From beginning to end, each recipe takes about 2 hrs. Most of this time, however, is rising and cooking time, during which you are free to do other things.

A few guidelines

FLOUR: If you want optimum results, the flour used must be fresh, so it is always best to buy flour in small quantities. I prefer unbleached white flour and plain stoneground wholemeal flour, and the ratio of the flours listed in the recipes can be adapted to suit your taste. You will find the various types of flour at supermarkets or in health-food stores.

SALT: A quantity of ½ tsp of salt is sufficient for one loaf, even though traditional recipes often suggest far more. In my view, adding any more salt is inappropriate.

SWEETNESS: A little sugar gives a softer flavour and sometimes helps to colour the bread, too. A quantity of 1 tbsp of sugar is quite enough for one loaf and in the following recipes I have suggested using either

Remember that leftovers of all kinds are great in sandwiches, whether you make your own bread or buy it.

When you are making bread, children can help by measuring all the ingredients.

honey or molasses. Molasses gives a lovely bitterness and a darker colour to the bread.

YEAST: Most people who make bread at home prefer to use fresh yeast, available from some bakers, health-food shops and supermarkets. It keeps for about two weeks in the refrigerator. After that time it loses its raising action and imparts an unpleasant, yeasty smell and taste to the bread. Old yeast becomes dark around the edges and sometimes develops a whitish film on it. Fresh yeast can also be stored in the freezer for about six months. Dry yeast gives good results. When using it, you need half the quantity that you would require of fresh yeast. A quantity of 30 g (1 oz) of fresh yeast will suffice for any quantity of flour up to 2 kg (4 lb 4 oz).

WATER: When making bread, the temperature of the water used is very important. If the water is too cold, the yeast is not activated, and if the water is too hot, the yeast is killed. The correct temperature is around 30°C/86°F. This is best achieved by mixing a ratio of two-thirds cold water from the tap with one-third boiling water from the kettle. When you dip your finger in the water it should be just warmer than lukewarm but not so hot as to burn. You should be able to touch it without discomfort. As various types of flour absorb water differently, the quantity of water indicated in the recipes is approximate. Sometimes the dough needs more moisture, sometimes less.

MIXING BOWL: A thick wooden mixing bowl, glass bowl or plastic bowl works better for making bread than a thin, metal bowl. A thick bowl keeps the heat in the dough better, and covering the bowl with a teatowel helps to hold the heat in while the dough is rising.

THE BREAD TIN: Bread cooks better in specially designed black bread tins than in any other type of tin. In all the recipes, I suggest using a standard loaf tin about 20 cm (8 in) long, which is obtainable from cookware shops and supermarkets. You can, of course, make bread rolls or any other shapes, using the recipes in this chapter.

KNEADING THE DOUGH: In the recipes, the bread is kneaded for about 2 mins after the bread has risen once. Recipes from other books may differ on this point but there is more than one way to make good bread. Knead by gently stretching (without tearing) the dough away from you with one hand and pulling the bottom half of the dough towards you with the other. Then with the heel of your hands fold the edges back in towards the centre, turn the dough a quarter turn and continue kneading in the same way. The dough soon becomes firmer and more elastic. Knead energetically. Once the dough has been kneaded and shaped to fit the tin, one of its sides is usually not completely smooth, as the folds you have made while kneading have formed a 'seam'. To obtain an attractively shaped bread, always position the dough in the bread tin with the seam underneath.

THE CRUST: To obtain a crust, brush the uncooked dough with a little lightly salted water or milk just before baking it. For a heightened golden colour, brush the top of the bread with beaten egg. To make the bread even more attractive and nutritious, sprinkle sesame seeds, poppy seeds, or wheatgerm on top of it before baking.

THE COOKING: The domestic oven is not quite as efficient as a specially designed baker's oven. Nevertheless, good results can be obtained at home. The oven must be preheated before baking begins, and the bread must be baked at a high temperature (220°C/ 450°F). Keep an eye on the cooking. Bake the bread in the centre of your oven. Most bread loaves take 35 to 40 mins to bake, but reduce the heat if the top of the bread begins to darken too much. Once the bread appears to be cooked, tip the loaf out onto a cake rack and check that it is cooked by tapping the bottom of the loaf; if it is cooked, it will make a hollow sound. If necessary, return it to the oven to cook a little more. The crust should be evenly browned on the sides and bottom.

Good luck! You will be impressed with your rapid progress in making bread.

Why not make bread rolls for a change? They cook more quickly than a large loaf and 'extras' will freeze well for later use.

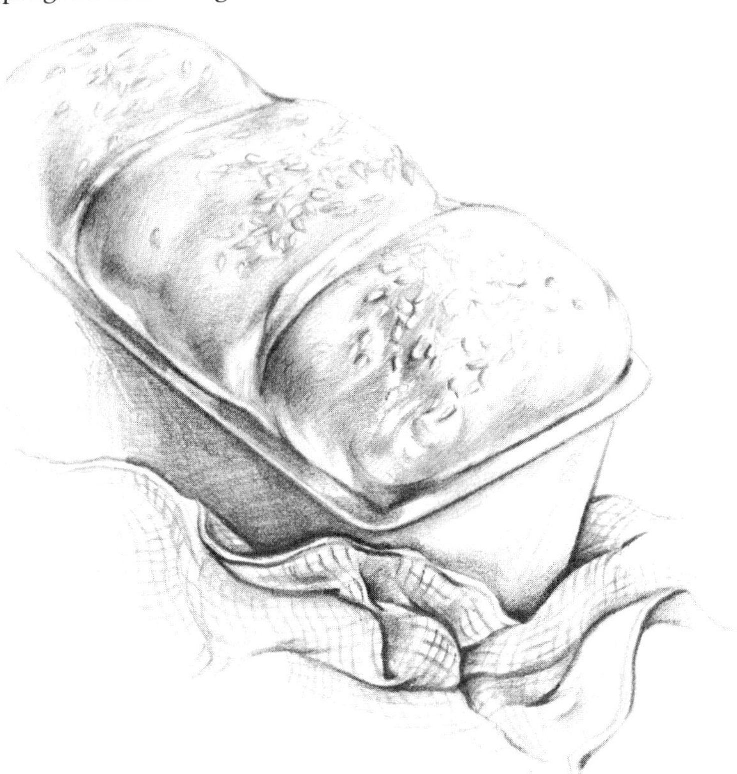

Multigrain loaf

This is a fun loaf to make. If you are trying this recipe for the first time, read the general information on bread before you begin. All the ingredients listed are obtainable in health-food shops and supermarkets. When preparing this loaf I usually use a bread tin about 20 cm (8 in) long.

MAKES 1 LOAF

3 tbsp wheat

3 tbsp unpearled barley

2 cups stoneground plain wholemeal flour

1 cup unbleached plain white flour

½ tsp salt

¼ cup linseeds (flaxseeds)

¼ cup sesame seeds

1 tbsp soy grits

1 tbsp polyunsaturated or light olive oil

1 tbsp honey

2 cups warm water (composed of cold tapwater and boiling water from the kettle)

30 g (1 oz) fresh yeast

Place wheat and unpearled barley in a saucepan, cover with water, bring to boil and boil for 10 mins. Drain and cool in cold water.

Place both types of flour, salt, linseeds, sesame seeds, soy grits, oil, honey and drained wheat and barley in a large, thick bowl.

Into a second bowl pour half of the warm water, crumble the yeast into the water and whisk until dissolved.

Using one hand, mix yeasty liquid into ingredients in large bowl, gradually incorporating remaining warm water (you may not need it all) until a soft dough forms and comes away from the sides of the bowl. It takes about 1 min. Cover with a teatowel and leave on the bench to rise for about 35 to 45 mins.

Remove dough from bowl and, using a little extra flour to prevent sticking, knead the dough energetically with both hands for about 2 mins. The dough quickly becomes firmer and more elastic.

Form dough into a sausage shape long enough to fit your oiled bread tin and place dough in tin with the seam underneath. The dough will fill about two-thirds of the tin. Again leave to rise until the dough almost reaches the rim of the tin. This takes about 20 mins.

Meanwhile, preheat oven to 220°C/450°F.

Bake bread in preheated oven for about 35 to 40 mins. Tip out onto a cake rack and check that the bread is cooked by tapping the bottom of the loaf. If it is cooked it will make a hollow sound. If necessary, return it to the oven to cook a little more.

Allow to cool before storing either in a flip-top bread container or in the cupboard in a brown paper bag.

Capsicum and leek loaf

This loaf is always popular for an alfresco lunch or barbecue and we use the dough also as a base for home-made pizza. The capsicum and leek may be cooked in advance to save time. If you are making this bread for the first time read the general information on bread in this chapter before you begin. When preparing this loaf I usually use a bread tin about 20 cm (8 in) long.

MAKES 1 LOAF

½ **red capsicum**

½ **green capsicum**

1 **tbsp olive oil**

1 **cup finely sliced leek**

3 **cups unbleached plain white flour**

1 **cup stoneground plain wholemeal flour**

1 **tsp curry powder**

½ **tsp salt**

½ **tbsp honey**

½ **cup chopped parsley**

1¾ **cups warm water (composed of cold tapwater and boiling water from the kettle)**

30 **g (1 oz) fresh yeast**

Remove seeds from capsicum. Wash and dice capsicum.

Heat olive oil in a saucepan and on low heat gently fry capsicum and leek for about 4 mins to soften them a little. Transfer to a plate to cool.

Place both types of flour, curry powder, salt and honey in a large, thick bowl and add cooled vegetables and parsley.

Into a second bowl pour half of the water, crumble yeast into water and whisk until dissolved.

Using one hand, gently mix yeasty liquid into ingredients in large bowl, gradually incorporating remaining warm water (you may not need it all) until a soft dough forms and comes away from the sides of the bowl. It takes about 1 min. Cover with a teatowel and leave on the bench to rise for 35 to 45 mins.

Remove dough from bowl and, using a little extra plain flour to prevent sticking, knead energetically with both hands for about 2 mins. The dough quickly becomes firmer and more elastic.

Form the dough into a sausage shape long enough to fit your oiled bread tin and place dough in tin with seam underneath. Again leave to rise until dough almost reaches the rim of the tin. It takes about 20 mins.

Meanwhile, preheat oven to 220°C/450°F.

Bake in preheated oven for about 35 to 40 mins. Tip out onto a cake rack and check that the bread is cooked by tapping the bottom of the loaf. If it is cooked it will make a hollow sound. If necessary, return it to the oven to cook a little more.

Allow to cool before storing either in a flip-top bread container or in the cupboard in a brown paper bag.

Mary's Irish soda bread

This bread, adapted from an Irish friend's recipe, is made without yeast and is, therefore, easy and quick to prepare. It is particularly popular served warm from the oven. If you wish, add a flavouring of your choice, such as chopped fresh herbs or a few caraway seeds.

MAKES 4 SMALL LOAVES

3 cups plain wholemeal flour

3 cups plain white flour

2 cups soy grit

2 tsp bicarbonate of soda

1 tbsp cream of tartar

1 tsp salt

2 tbsp sugar

3 tbsp peanut oil

about 2½ cups low-fat milk

Preheat oven to 250°C/500°F.

In a large bowl mix the two types of flour, soy grit, bicarbonate of soda, cream of tartar, salt and sugar. Make a hollow in the centre and pour the oil and half of the milk into it. Using one hand, mix oil and milk with flour, gradually adding the remaining milk until a dough forms. You may either not need all of the milk or you may not have quite enough, depending on the quality of your flour.

Place dough on a floured bench and form it into a ball.

Lightly dust a baking sheet with flour and place the dough in the centre of the baking sheet. Flatten it a little and cut it into quarters. Sprinkle the top with a little flour and cook in the preheated oven for 30–35 mins. The bread will be brown and crusty. Reduce temperature during the last 5 mins if the top of the loaf starts to brown too much.

Coleslaw and avocado sandwich

The mixed shredded cabbage and carrot used here are excellent sources of vitamins, fibre and other good things. When including avocado in a sandwich, I find it unnecessary to spread the bread with butter or margarine.

SERVES 1

½ small avocado

a few drops lemon juice

1 or 2 drops tabasco sauce

freshly ground black pepper

2 tbsp finely shredded cabbage

2 tbsp finely grated carrot

2 slices wholegrain, wholemeal or rye bread

Mash avocado with lemon juice, tabasco and a little pepper, then mix in shredded cabbage and grated carrot. Spoon this preparation onto one slice of bread and cover with the other slice. Cut sandwich in half and enjoy it.

Egg and salad wholemeal sandwich

This satisfying sandwich is quick to prepare, especially if you have a hard-boiled egg on hand. The addition of butter or margarine is unnecessary if you spread the mashed egg on the bread first. Remember to limit your consumption of eggs to about 3 to 4 per week per person.

SERVES 1

1 small egg

a pinch of curry powder (optional)

freshly ground black pepper

2 slices wholegrain bread

1 large lettuce leaf, finely shredded

2 slices cooked beetroot

1 small carrot, grated

Place egg in a saucepan of cold water, bring to boil, cover pan, turn off heat and leave for 15 mins. Transfer egg to cold water to cool if you wish.

Mash egg and season with curry powder and a little pepper. Spread egg on both slices of bread and top one side with lettuce, beetroot and grated carrot. Cover with the other slice of bread, cut sandwich in half and enjoy it.

Tuna and vegetable pizza

This recipe was created with Phillip, a friend who runs a pizza place and cares about the health of his clients. For the pizza base, stop at your baker or pizza shop and buy a little dough. Keep the dough in the refrigerator until required: for a few hours, if necessary. Two large pizza platters about 25 cm (about 10 in) in diameter will be required.

MAKES 2 LARGE PIZZAS

about 1 kg (about 2 lb) bread dough from the baker (preferably wholemeal)

6 tbsp bottled or home-made Italian tomato sauce (chapter 7)

150 g (5 oz) grated low-fat mozzarella cheese

12 button mushrooms, finely sliced

a 300 g (11 oz) can tuna, drained

1 green capsicum, halved and finely sliced

a 400 g (14 oz) can corn kernels (no added salt), drained

2 tbsp pepitas

12 pitted black olives, halved

Cut dough in half and form it into two smooth balls. Roll out the two balls of dough to the size of your pizza platters. Place dough in oiled platters.

Preheat oven to 220°C/450°F.

To garnish pizza bases, first spread tomato sauce evenly over dough then on top sprinkle half of the cheese and all the mushroom, tuna, capsicum, corn, pepitas and the halved black olives. Sprinkle with remaining cheese and cook in preheated oven until pizza base is dry and lightly browned underneath (this takes from 15 to 20 mins). Turn pizzas around and interchange the platters during cooking to allow for even cooking (if necessary, lower temperature during cooking).

Buon appetito!

Vegetarian pizza

This fast home-made pizza uses a base of bread dough that you can obtain at your local baker or pizza shop. Keep the dough in the refrigerator (for a few hours if necessary) until required. The topping of this pizza can be changed according to taste. Cut the vegetables very finely. Sometimes a little juice may escape from the vegetables during the cooking, so just pour it off before cutting and serving the pizza. For this pizza too you will need two large pizza platters about 25 cm (about 10 in) in diameter. It is illustrated opposite page 53.

MAKES 2 LARGE PIZZAS

about 1 kg (about 2 lb) bread dough from the baker (preferably wholemeal)

6 tbsp bottled or home-made Italian tomato sauce (chapter 7)

150 g (about 5 oz) grated low-fat mozzarella cheese

18 button mushrooms, finely sliced

1 medium zucchini, finely sliced

1 small green capsicum, halved and finely sliced

1 small red capsicum, halved and finely sliced

a 400 g (14 oz) can corn kernels (no added salt), drained

2 tbsp pepitas

12 pitted black olives, halved

Cut dough in half and form it into two smooth balls. Roll out the two balls of pastry to the size of your pizza platters. Place dough in oiled platters.

Preheat oven to 220°C/450°F.

To garnish pizza bases, first spread tomato sauce evenly over dough, then on top sprinkle half of the cheese and all the mushroom, zucchini, capsicum, corn, pepitas and the halved black olives. Sprinkle with remaining cheese and cook in preheated oven until pizza base is dry and lightly browned underneath (this takes 15 to 20 mins). Turn pizzas around and interchange the platters during cooking to allow for even cooking (if necessary, lower temperature during cooking).

Well Dressed and Well Seasoned

It is true that many of us today do not have as much time to devote to preparing meals as we would like to have. Yet we are concerned about our health and want to eat good food. Remember, often the best food is also the easiest to prepare. In this chapter you will find sauces and dressings that can be made quickly and can turn vegetables or simple grilled meat or fish into an imaginative meal. You will see what a difference the use of herbs and spices can make to your cooking, in a surprisingly short time. Speed and simplicity do not mean you have to lose out on flavour or goodness.

A seasoning should enhance the natural flavour of the main ingredients of the dish, and it is interesting to note the various seasonings used throughout the countries of the world. People in hot climates generally use pungent seasonings, and even within a country there is enormous variation in the ways food is flavoured. Those living beside the sea have a higher threshold for salt and so use more salty seasonings in general than those living inland. In southern Europe, cooks use olive oil and garlic, while in the north it is traditional to cook with butter and shallots. There are many such examples.

If a particular seasoning does not reflect the traditions or geographical characteristics of a place, it must certainly reflect the habits, tastes and knowledge of the cook. I have learnt a lot about balancing flavour by learning to prepare dishes from many different countries, and by gradually increasing the use of herbs and spices in my cooking I have been able to reduce the amount of fat and salt I use. It is good to know that a dish that is composed of ingredients having different shapes and textures offers greater contrast on the palate and, therefore, needs less seasoning than a plainer dish.

In the various chapters of this book you will find new and tantalising ways of using herbs and spices. If fresh herbs are unavailable, a smaller quantity of dried herbs can be substituted.

It is important to remember to use cooking fat and seasoning fat such as oils, margarine and butter in moderation. Most oils and fats are nearly 100 per cent fat so they supply equivalent amounts of energy (kilojoules). Standard table margarines and butter contain some water, and the fat-reduced varieties are processed with higher water levels.

We should reduce the *total* amount of fat in our diets and, in particular, saturated fats found mostly in fatty meat, butter, cream, and dairy foods that have not had the fat reduced. Foods made with these ingredients such as pastries, biscuits and cakes are often high in saturated fat also. It is sensible to use low-fat milk, cheeses and yoghurt. Mono-unsaturated oil, such as olive oil, and polyunsaturated oils, including most vegetable oils such as sunflower, safflower and peanut oil, are preferred for cooking, as they seem less likely to increase the level of fats in the blood. A high blood fat level is a risk factor for heart disease.

The excessive use of salt and salty ingredients, like soy sauce, is also of some concern in regard to high blood pressure. It is easy to reduce the use of salt to a minimum by seasoning food with fresh, flavoursome ingredients and making sure there is a contrast of shape and texture within a dish. A clever cook uses seasonings such as lemon juice, spices, pepper in particular, and herbs, especially parsley, which is always available. In our family cooking we have reduced our use of salt dramatically. I add a little salt to the cooking water for plain pasta, rice or potatoes, and I also use it when making bread.

A few herbs from the garden, snipped over pasta, into soup, or onto salads and meats, can add instant flavour.

Salad dressing

The purpose of a dressing is to create harmony and a little moisture and flavour among the ingredients, to give them a common note. More often than not, salads are overdressed. This mistake can turn a beautiful salad into an unnecessarily fatty dish. If the salad ingredients are well dried, 1 to 2 tbsp of dressing is all that is required for about four people, and the easiest way to dry green leaves such as lettuce is to use a salad spinner, a must in any kitchen. At the final moment a salad likes to be gently and thoroughly tossed.

It is much more fun to make your own salad dressing, which tastes better than the commercial ones and gives you the pleasure of stamping your own touch on the salad. I would particularly like to draw your attention to the flexibility of a yoghurt dressing to replace rich dressings such as mayonnaise. Simply mix a little low-fat natural yoghurt with lemon juice or vinegar and season with spices or herbs of your choice. You will find it very satisfying trying something new.

Experiment with various types of vinegar and oils, too. Walnut oil is delicious for a special occasion and olive oil is appropriate for all Mediterranean–style salads that contain ingredients such as tomato, capsicum, greens, olives and fish. If you find the flavour of pure olive oil a little strong try the light olive oil, which has a milder flavour. At home we use peanut oil in salads in which we want to keep the taste of the dressing fairly neutral. Variety is the spice of life!

French dressing with mustard and peanut oil

This is the dressing that many French families prepare for the almost daily green salad, which is served after the main course. Occasionally a little chopped garlic is added to it.

SERVES 4

a pinch of salt

freshly ground black pepper

½ tsp hot mustard

1 tsp red wine vinegar

3 tsp peanut oil

In a small bowl place salt, a little pepper and mustard. Stir in vinegar and, lastly, add oil. Stir well, taste and add a little more vinegar or oil if necessary.

Tomato and dill dressing

This delicate dressing will add instant flavour to warm vegetables, and poached or grilled fish. If you wish, you can warm the dressing a little, and the dill can be replaced by another herb.

SERVES ABOUT 4

1 large tomato or 2 small ones

2 tsp red wine vinegar

1–1½ tbsp olive oil

½ finely chopped white onion or 1 shallot

2 tbsp finely cut dill

freshly ground black pepper

Trim core of tomato, place tomato in a bowl and cover with boiling water. After 10 secs, remove from bowl and dip tomato in cold water. Peel and halve tomato and gently squeeze out seeds. Dice tomato.

In a bowl combine diced tomato, red wine vinegar, oil, onion and dill, and season with a little pepper.

Mediterranean dressing

Mediterranean dressing may vary from one country to another but good olive oil remains the common ingredient. The acidity is provided by either lemon juice or vinegar, and various condiments such as peppers, onions or herbs are added for extra zest. The selection of ingredients is a question of taste and imagination.

SERVES ABOUT 4

juice of ½ lemon
freshly ground black pepper
¼ tsp dried oregano
1 tbsp olive oil
½ tbsp chopped onion

In a small bowl thoroughly mix lemon juice, a little pepper, oregano and, lastly, olive oil and onion.

Taste and if necessary add more lemon juice and/or oil to balance the flavour.

If you must prepare a dressing well in advance, add the chopped onion just before using the dressing.

Minted cucumber and yoghurt dressing

This dressing particularly suits salads consisting of raw or cooked vegetables, such as celery, radishes and beans, and goes well with barbecues.

SERVES 4

a 10 cm (4 in) piece of cucumber
juice of ½ lemon
1 tsp mint
½ clove garlic, chopped
½ cup low-fat natural yoghurt

Peel, halve and seed cucumber and dice finely. Mix well with lemon juice, mint, garlic and yoghurt, and refrigerate until required.

Creamy coriander and pine nut dressing

This peppery hot dressing can be whirled together in a food processor in no time at all and is very versatile. It is delicious with cold fish, vegetables, pasta, and salads based on pulses.

SERVES ABOUT 4

½ cup fresh coriander leaves
1 tbsp pine nuts
1 tbsp low-fat natural yoghurt
1 tbsp low-fat milk
¼ tsp hot chilli paste or a pinch of chilli powder

In a food processor blend coriander, pine nuts, yoghurt, milk and chilli paste to a purée.

If you don't have a food processor, chop coriander and pine nuts finely and mix well with yoghurt, milk and chilli paste. Refrigerate until required.

Spicy Asian dressing

This dressing goes best with salads of finely sliced vegetables, such as cabbage and spinach, or even bean sprouts. Avoid serving this dressing to young children as the chilli is too hot for them. The dressing tastes better when made at the last moment.

SERVES ABOUT 4

½ tsp sesame oil

juice of 1 lime or 1 small lemon

1 tsp salt-reduced soy sauce

1 tsp peanut or polyunsaturated oil

1 small chilli

½ clove garlic

1 tbsp fresh coriander leaves or 1 tbsp flat-leaved parsley

In a bowl combine sesame oil, lime juice, soy sauce and oil.

Slice chilli very finely.

Peel and chop garlic.

Stir chilli, garlic and coriander leaves into dressing.

Almost mayonnaise

This cold sauce resembles a mayonnaise in both appearance and flavour and is made using low-fat soft cheese with a milk-fat content of less than 8 per cent. The result is not too cheesy, and the smooth sauce contains less than one-third of the calories of traditional mayonnaise made with oil.

SERVES ABOUT 4

3 tbsp quark (fresh low-fat soft cheese with a milk-fat content of less than 8 per cent)

1 egg

½ tsp hot English mustard

1 tbsp low-fat milk

a small pinch of salt

freshly ground black pepper

Take cheese out of refrigerator to bring it to room temperature.

Bring a small saucepan of water to the boil and cook egg for 7 to 8 mins. Remove egg and refresh in cold water for about 10 secs before peeling it while it is still warm. Halve egg and place warm yolk in an electric blender (keep the white for a salad or sandwich for lunch). Add mustard, milk, soft cheese, salt and a little pepper. Blend to a smooth creamy consistency. Place in a serving bowl or refrigerate if not using within 1 hr.

SERVING SUGGESTION: Serve with salads, cold meats, fish, vegetables, and so on.

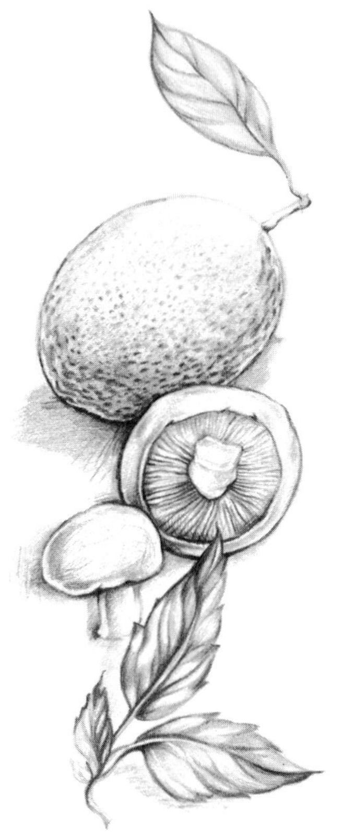

If a vegetable sauce is a little too sweet, add a few drops of lemon juice and/or a spice such as freshly ground black pepper or chilli pepper.

Minimum effort, maximum effect – and taste! Atlantic salmon (page 93) with crisp vegetables and tangy vegetable sauce (page 87)

The joys of sauces

Many inexperienced cooks believe sauces are difficult and slow to make. On the contrary, sauces are time-savers – they can add almost instant flavour and style to the most simple meal. If your repertoire includes some of the following sauces, you will always be able to prepare a meal with flair, even if you are pressed for time.

In professional kitchens the last position you usually hold before becoming an executive chef is chef in charge of sauces, and for many chefs this is the favourite post of all. Making sauces gives great joy to the cook. A sauce's smoothness coats the palate, creating a full flavour experience, and it provides moisture for other foods. In the cooking of yesteryear, smoothness was obtained by binding a sauce with butter and flour mixed together, or by adding cream. Nowadays, we know that these ingredients, although delicious, must be used in moderation and this has encouraged cooks all over the world to look for alternatives, while still retaining the rich texture and flavour of the sauce. Thanks to the invention of the electric food processor, we can now make the finest vegetable purées to give richness to soups and sauces. Best of all, these can often be made in a few minutes.

In the following recipes you will discover low-fat ways of making sauces, but I have not gone to extremes and eliminated fat completely. Every cook benefits greatly by learning to prepare a range of sauces, like the Italian tomato sauce that can be served with so many foods from pasta to vegetables, fish and meats; the curry sauce to serve with more exotic preparations; or a simple vegetable sauce, such as the pea and cummin sauce to accompany a pan-fried chicken breast or a grilled fish fillet.

I find it useful to have a little chicken stock permanently on hand in my freezer for making vegetable sauces, and by using vegetables and your favourite spices and herbs, you can create the most original sauces. Remember that pumpkin and carrot are sweeter than celery and leek. If a sauce is too sweet, add a little lemon juice or dry wine for acidity, or even some chopped herbs. Spices can also impart a desired bitterness.

Practise a few of the sauces and you will soon become a fast and confident sauce cook.

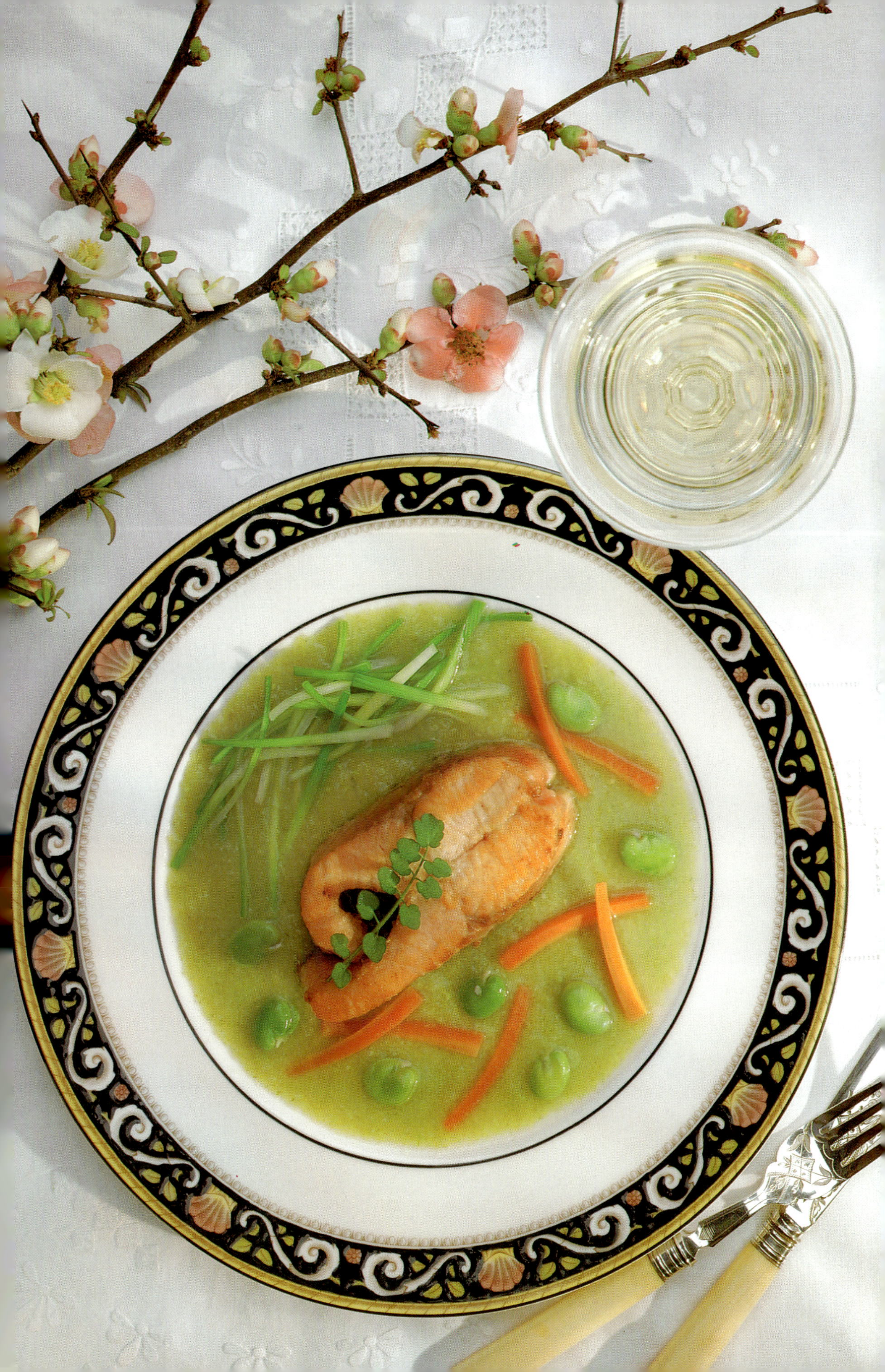

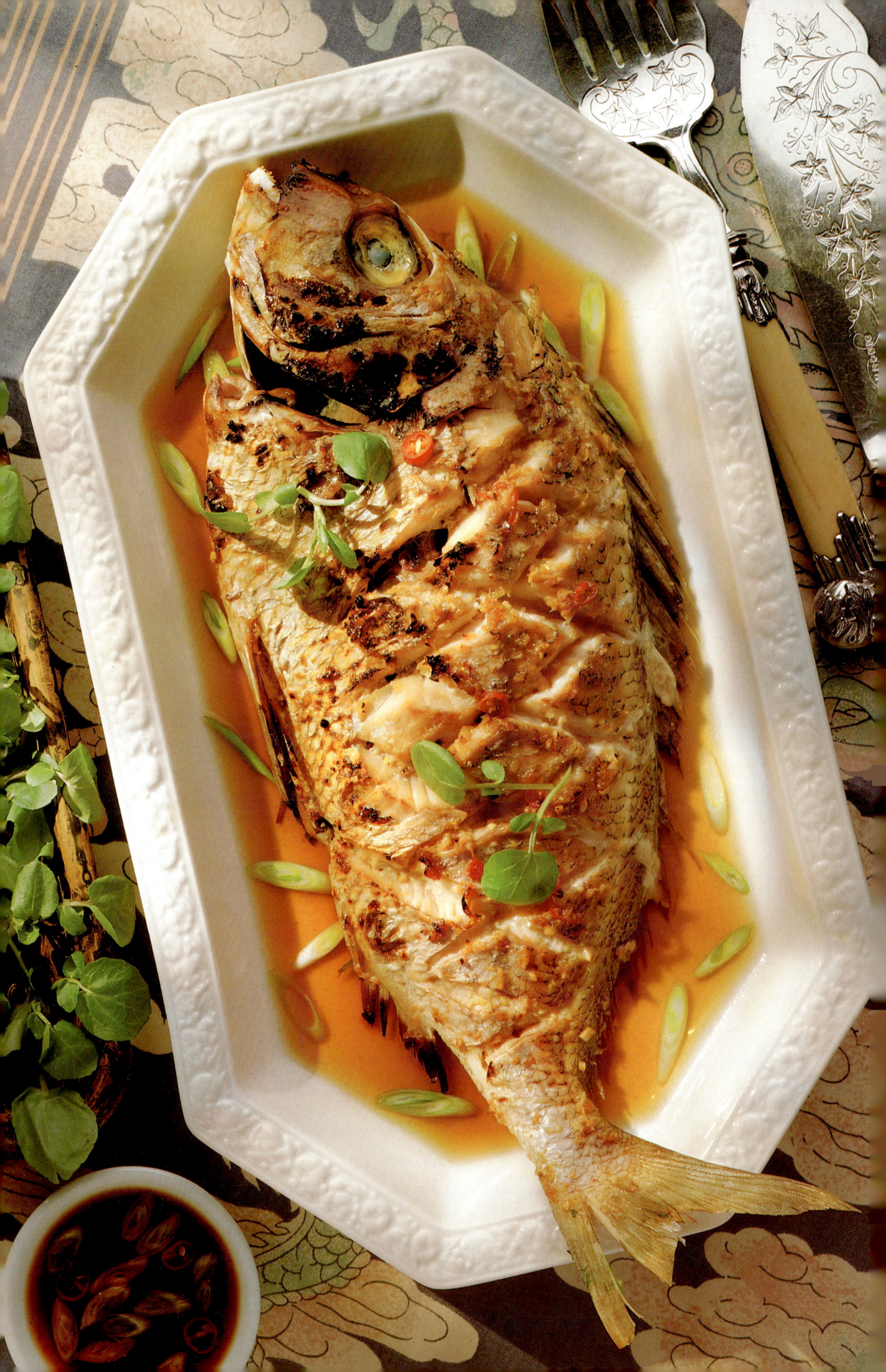

Italian tomato sauce

The tomato is an extraordinary ingredient whose soft, sweet, rich texture makes it extremely versatile. This Italian-style tomato sauce can be used with pasta, fish, vegetables, meat, pancakes and pizzas. I find it just as easy to make double the quantity and freeze what is not required. It is ideal to have on hand if we need a very quick midweek meal, or if friends call unexpectedly.

SERVES ABOUT 4

6 medium ripe tomatoes

½ medium brown onion

1 stick celery, from the heart

1 medium carrot

2 sprigs parsley or 1 sprig basil or 1 small sprig thyme

1 clove garlic

freshly ground black pepper

1 tsp olive oil (optional)

Cut all vegetables into small pieces and place in a saucepan with herbs, garlic and a little pepper. Cook on medium heat for 20 to 30 mins.

Remove herbs and pass vegetables through a mouli or fine strainer, or leave unstrained if you prefer a chunky sauce. Check seasoning and stir in oil before serving sauce hot. If you wish, you can also add more pepper and freshly chopped herbs like basil, tarragon or coriander.

Quick mushroom and basil sauce

This mushroom sauce can be served with pasta, chicken, chops or vegetables and can also be served as a vegetable dish on its own.

SERVES ABOUT 2

100 g (3½ oz) mushrooms

1 clove garlic

2 tomatoes

1 tsp olive oil

1 tbsp finely sliced basil leaves

freshly ground black pepper

a few drops lemon juice

Briefly wash mushrooms in a large quantity of cold water. Slice mushrooms finely.

Peel and chop garlic.

Halve and chop tomatoes finely.

In a large frying pan heat oil. When oil is hot fry mushroom on high heat for about 2 mins. Add garlic, stir well then add tomato. Bring to boil and boil for 3 mins. Stir in basil and season with a little pepper and lemon juice.

◁

The freshest fish, brushed with a spicy Asian marinade and baked whole. Delicious, quick cuisine (page 96)

Leek and green pea sauce

This sauce is quick to prepare and ideally served with poached white meats such as chicken and turkey, or with steamed vegetables. It is a tasty substitute for butter, cream or rich sauces.

SERVES 4–6

1 small leek or ½ a large one

¼ brown onion

a little peanut or polyunsaturated oil

1 tbsp white vinegar

1½ cups chicken stock (chapter 7) or water

about ½ cup shelled peas

freshly ground black pepper

a pinch of nutmeg

Cut leek in four lengthwise, leaving the root intact. Wash leek thoroughly in lukewarm water to remove grit, then slice it thinly.

Peel and finely chop onion.

Brush a saucepan with oil and cook leek and onion on low heat for a few minutes, stirring regularly to avoid burning.

Add vinegar and chicken stock, and bring to boil before adding peas. Cook until peas are soft.

Blend vegetables and liquid to a fine runny purée, adding extra water if necessary to obtain a sauce consistency.

Before serving season with a little pepper and nutmeg, or other spices and herbs of your choice.

Pea and cummin sauce

This sauce is perfect with pan-fried meat such as a chicken breast or loin of lamb. When your meat is cooked, transfer it to a plate and keep it warm, then reheat sauce in the same pan. The sauce also goes well with vegetables, rice, potatoes or pasta, and is easy to make.

SERVES 4–6

1 tomato, finely diced

½ tsp of ground cummin

¼ brown onion, finely chopped

1 small carrot

½ cup shelled peas

1½ cups chicken stock (chapter 7) or water

a pinch of cayenne pepper

In a medium saucepan place tomato, cummin and onion and cook gently on medium heat for 2 mins.

Peel and finely slice carrot and add to pan. Add peas and chicken stock, bring to boil and cook for about 10 mins until carrots are tender.

In a food processor blend vegetables and liquid to a very smooth sauce and strain it, if you wish.

Stir in cayenne pepper just before serving.

Tangy vegetable sauce

This sauce is beautiful with fish or chicken and even with vegetables, such as artichokes and asparagus. The sauce needs to be blended to a very smooth purée and then strained.

SERVES ABOUT 4

1 tbsp chopped onion

½ cup dry white wine

½ cup finely sliced celery

½ cup finely sliced leek

1 cup water

a small pinch of salt

freshly ground black pepper

1 tsp polyunsaturated margarine or butter

a few drops lemon juice

Place onion and white wine in a small saucepan and simmer until most of the liquid has evaporated. Add celery and leek and stir for 2 or 3 mins before adding water, salt and pepper. Bring to boil, cover and cook until vegetables are soft.

Blend vegetables and liquid to a very fine purée then strain through a fine strainer. Return sauce to pan and put aside until required.

Before serving, reheat sauce and whisk in margarine. Season with a few drops of lemon juice.

Anytime curry sauce

You can adapt a curry sauce to suit your mood, or to suit the ingredients with which it will be served, by adding spices, such as fennel with fish, cummin with pulses, or herbs, such as coriander with fish and vegetables, or parsley with almost anything. At the end of this recipe is my recipe for curry powder. I hope you will try it.

SERVES ABOUT 4

½ brown onion

a 2 cm (¾ in) piece of ginger

2 cloves garlic

4 tomatoes

2 tsp peanut oil

4 fennel seeds

10 cummin seeds

2 tsp curry powder

½ tsp hot chilli paste (optional)

1 tbsp desiccated coconut (optional) or 1 tbsp finely sliced fresh coriander leaves (optional)

Peel onion, ginger and garlic then blend them to a fine purée. Alternatively, chop them finely.

Halve and chop tomatoes finely.

In a medium saucepan place oil, fennel seeds, cummin seeds and puréed onion, ginger and garlic. Cook on low heat for at least 5 mins while stirring with a wooden spoon. If ingredients start to burn add 1 or 2 tbsp of water. Add curry powder and stir for about 1 min before adding tomato. Bring to a simmer and cook on low heat for about 10 mins, stirring occasionally.

About 1 min before serving, stir in chilli paste, desiccated coconut or coriander.

SERVING SUGGESTION: Serve with steamed vegetables, with pan-fried or steamed fish, with chicken or with rice.

CURRY POWDER: Grind to a powder 4 tbsp coriander seeds, 1¼ tbsp cummin seeds, 1 tbsp fenugreek seeds, 1½ tbsp turmeric, 1 tbsp black peppercorns, 6 dried chillies and 10 cardamom seeds. Blend the spices together well (you get about ¾ cup) and store in an airtight jar away from sunlight.

Pesto sauce

This is the classic Italian sauce made with basil, a very aromatic herb. One teaspoon of pesto is sufficient to season a dish of vegetables for four, and mixed in a vegetable soup, it does wonders! Of course, its most common use is in pasta and salads. Pesto sauce keeps well in a jar in the fridge for several weeks. Flatten the top of your leftover pesto and add a little olive oil to seal the sauce and prevent it from oxidising. Alternatively, it may be frozen. This famous sauce can be made in minutes.

MAKES ABOUT 1 CUP

about 1 cup basil leaves

2 tbsp pine nuts

3 cloves garlic, peeled

2 tbsp grated parmesan cheese or 1 tbsp grated pecorino and 1 tbsp grated parmesan cheese

2 tbsp olive oil

Check that all basil leaves are unblemished. Wash basil, drain well and dry briefly in a clean teatowel.

In a food processor, place basil, pine nuts, garlic and parmesan cheese and blend to a paste. Add oil and blend until well incorporated.

Peanut sauce

This sauce is particularly handy if you are vegetarian, as nuts are a source of protein. It goes well with vegetable kebabs and other vegetarian dishes, and is also delicious with fish or meat kebabs. Many health-food shops and nut shops sell freshly made peanut butter with no added salt.

SERVES 4

a 2 cm (¾ in) piece of ginger

½ small onion

1 clove garlic

¾ cup water

3 tbsp desiccated coconut

1 tsp peanut oil

½ tsp curry powder

2 tsp Asian fish sauce or salt-reduced soy sauce

1½ tbsp crunchy peanut butter (no added salt)

½ tsp hot chilli paste

Blend ginger, onion and garlic to a purée or chop them finely.

Place ¾ cup water in a saucepan with coconut and bring to boil for 30 secs. Turn off heat and allow the coconut to infuse the liquid.

Gently fry the onion mixture in oil in a small saucepan on low heat for 5 mins, stirring with a wooden spoon to prevent burning. Add curry powder and fish sauce, and stir well before adding peanut butter and chilli paste.

Strain coconut liquid into a bowl, pressing coconut to extract as much flavour as possible. Add liquid to peanut sauce and stir thoroughly until the sauce is smooth. Cook on low heat for 2 mins, then serve.

Creamy savoury topping

This is the low-fat preparation to enjoy with baked potatoes or other savoury dishes such as steamed asparagus, and it acts as a substitute for sour cream, cream or butter. The addition of herbs, such as snipped chives or chopped parsley, or grated orange or lemon rind is also lovely, and the recipe takes no time to prepare.

SERVES 4–6

3 tbsp low-fat natural yoghurt

5 tbsp quark (fresh low-fat soft cheese with a milk-fat content of less than 8 per cent)

1 tbsp low-fat milk

freshly ground black pepper

2 pinches of cayenne pepper or paprika

juice of ½ lemon

Blend all ingredients until smooth and refrigerate until required.

Chicken stock

Chicken stock is a very handy preparation to have ready in the freezer and can help to make a fast and flavoursome sauce or soup on another occasion. When the stock is made and not used immediately, boil it down to a small quantity, cool it and freeze it in a small container. Mark the container to show the contents and date, and use the stock within about three months.

MAKES ABOUT 8 CUPS

about 1 kg (about 2 lb) chicken bones (carcass, neck, wings, with skin and fat removed)

12 cups water

1 carrot, sliced

1 onion, sliced

1 stick celery or a piece of leek, sliced

5 black peppercorns, crushed

1 clove

a few sprigs parsley, 1 small sprig thyme, ½ bay leaf, washed and tied together with kitchen string

Place chicken bones and water in a large saucepan. Bring to boil and skim surface of liquid to remove foam. Add all ingredients and simmer for about 1 hr, skimming surface again if necessary. Strain stock, discard bones and vegetables and allow to cool before storing. Remove any fat from surface.

To make a flavoursome broth or soup, a whole chicken can be simmered in water with carrot, celery, onion, leeks, and so on. The delicious poached chicken will provide the main course for your family dinner, leaving the stock for use another time.

A Kettle of Fish

Fish is fantastic for cooks in a hurry – especially those concerned about their health. It is easy to prepare and can be either a simple family meal or, with an unusual sauce or distinctive seasoning, a special-occasion dish. Long before we human beings learned to cultivate vegetables or domesticate animals, fish was an important part of our diet. This is not so surprising when we know that humans first evolved at the edge of rivers, seas and lakes. For centuries fish was cheaper than bread in most parts of the world and apparently in the seventeenth century in Scotland, salmon, that exquisite pink fish that nowadays costs about $25 per kilogram in Australia, was so common that a law was passed to stop employers from giving it to their servants more than three times a week. Perhaps they ate pike on the other four days.

No doubt most of you have heard about the benefits of eating fish regularly. Well-cooked fish is light and easy to digest as well as being an excellent source of protein, vitamins and calcium. These benefits are partly negated if the fish is battered, crumbed and fried, or served with a rich sauce. Most of our fish are low in fat, though fish contains the special type of fatty acids known as Omega-3, which may help lower blood fats, reduce blood pressure and prevent the blood from clotting too readily – good reasons for including fish regularly in our diets.

Shopping for fish

The price of fish varies according to its availability and the demand for it. The weather plays an important role, as bad weather can prevent fishermen from harvesting. Contrary to what many people think, a cheap fish can be an excellent buy. For instance, my local fishmonger has sardines and flathead on sale at budget prices for most of the week. From my experience, the better fish shops are the busiest ones, and I have noticed when visiting a market for the first time that the busiest shop sells the freshest and usually the cheapest fish.

It is worthwhile becoming friendly with your fishmonger, who will then recognise you when you shop. Shopkeepers love familiar faces and look after them better.

Learn to identify fish by their names and share your knowledge with your children. In a good fish shop you will always see a fair selection of whole fish, attractively displayed. Try fish that you are not familiar with. All fish is good when fresh. A fresh fish looks wet and firm and has shiny, slippery skin with scales that hold together closely. The eyes are usually clear and bulging and the gills are pink or dark red. An unfresh fish appears flaccid, for it has lost its firmness. The scales are loose and often dry, and the smell is offputting, to say the least!

Even when I need fish fillets I prefer to choose a whole fish and ask the fishmonger to fillet it for me; but remember, a filleted fish loses its freshness more quickly than a whole fish. A dedicated fishmonger will prepare the fish the way you require it, whether it be simply cleaned, scaled and filleted, cut into cutlets, or just skinned. You may also ask to take away the bones and heads of the fish you purchase for use in a soup or stock.

If you are unable to make up your mind, ask the fishmonger for advice. Explain what you want to use the fish for and how many people you intend to serve.

Your fishmonger will appreciate some feedback about your previous purchase, such as, 'We enjoyed that gurnard so much last week'. Selling fish is a very hard and demanding job and any encouragement helps considerably.

Cooking fish

The following recipes illustrate various simple and quick ways of cooking fish. Whichever technique you use, the fish flesh will change colour as it cooks, from a

When grilling fish, place it about 3 to 5 cm (1½ to 2½ in) from the heat.

raw translucence to a whitish-pink or light-brown colour, depending on the type of fish. A well-cooked fish is moist and the flesh flakes easily. To check if it is cooked, probe a whole fish or fillet at its thickest part using the blade of a small knife. If the blade meets no resistance, the fish is ready. When cooking fish, whether whole, cutlets or fillets, use a long, wide spatula to turn or lift it. When baking or pan-frying, use a tray or frying pan just large enough to hold the fish; otherwise the fat or liquid used or the natural juices from the fish will burn in the extra space.

You will find some helpful cookery hints in the introductions to each recipe. And remember, for most cooks, it takes more than one attempt before being totally satisfied with the result of a dish.

Pan-fried fish fillets with spices

Take your time to choose a very fresh fish just the size you need, and ask your fishmonger to scale and fillet it for you. You may wish to ask to take the bones home for use in a stock later. This dish can be cooked in a flash.

SERVES 2

a 500 g (about 1 lb) fish, filleted

1 tsp paprika

freshly ground black pepper

a pinch of cummin seeds

a little olive oil

juice of ½ lemon

Dry the fish fillets and season them with paprika, a little black pepper and cummin seeds, evenly spread over fish.

Brush a heavy frying pan with olive oil. Heat pan and when hot, place fillets in pan, skinless side facing down, and cook the first side for 2 to 4 mins, depending on thickness. Refrain from moving fish around during cooking. Using a flat spatula, turn fish and cook second side, adding a little more oil if really necessary.

Probe fillet with the tip of a knife blade. If it goes through easily the fish is cooked.

Squeeze lemon juice over fish when it is still in pan, and serve immediately.

SERVING SUGGESTION: Serve with Asian noodles or brown rice, and a mixed salad.

Australian grilled fish fillets

Cooking fish this way is popular with Australian families. In France the average stove or oven is not equipped with a griller, so we tend to pan-fry instead. When grilling, avoid placing the fish too close to the flame or heat, and be careful not to place it too far away. A distance of 3 to 5 cm (1½ to 2½ in) is advisable, and the thinner the fillet, the closer it can be to the heat. Select one or two fresh fish and ask your fishmonger to scale and fillet them for you. Use cutlets instead of fillets, if you wish.

SERVES 4

4 pieces of fish fillet about 150 g (5 oz) each (e.g. silver trevally, perch, barramundi)

a little plain flour

freshly ground black pepper

1 tsp paprika or curry powder or a spice of your choice

a little olive oil

4 lemon wedges

Lightly coat well-dried fish fillets with a little flour seasoned with black pepper and paprika.

Set grill at medium heat.

Brush a baking sheet with a little olive oil, place fish on sheet and put under grill. When the top of the fish starts to brown, turn fillets using a flat spatula. When the second side has started to brown, check if fish is cooked by probing it with the blade of a knife. If it goes through easily the fish is ready. Serve immediately with lemon wedges.

SERVING SUGGESTION: Serve with brown rice or steamed potatoes and seasonal vegetables.

Pan-fried Atlantic salmon cutlet

Tasmanian Atlantic salmon is one of the most beautiful fish available to us in Australia and is a treat for special occasions. Because it is a meaty fish, about 120 g (4 oz) is sufficient per person. As the texture of salmon is very delicate, ensure that the fishmonger cuts it on the spot and does not give you precut cutlets. Ocean trout is a good substitute for Atlantic salmon and is a little cheaper. This very special dish is shown opposite page 84.

SERVES 2

2 Atlantic salmon cutlets or 1 large one

a little plain flour

freshly ground black pepper

½ tbsp olive oil

juice of ½ lemon

Very lightly coat the well-dried cutlets with plain flour and season with pepper.

Heat oil in a frying pan that is just the right size for two cutlets. Gently place cutlets in pan and cook on high heat for 1 min before reducing to medium heat and cooking for a further 2 mins. Gently turn fish and cook the second side for about 3 mins. When the fish is ready, the flesh can be easily detached from the bone at the centre. Squeeze a few drops of lemon over fish while it is still in pan and serve.

SERVING SUGGESTION: Serve with small or finely cut steamed vegetables and a tangy vegetable sauce (chapter 7).

Steamed fish fillets al pesto

Having a large steamer is a great help in the kitchen and a wide range of steamers is available in department stores, cookware shops and Chinese grocery stores. Ideally, the food to be steamed should be placed on a plate in the steamer so that the plate collects any delicious juices that escape during cooking. If you have no time to make your own pesto sauce or if basil is not in season, you may like to use one of the commercial pesto sauces, some of which are good.

SERVES 2

2 pieces of fish fillet, 150 g (5 oz) each

freshly ground black pepper

2 tsp pesto sauce (chapter 7)

Bring about 2 cups of water in steamer to boil.

Place fish, skin down, on a plate and season with a little freshly ground black pepper. Place plate in steamer, cover and cook for 4 to 8 mins, depending on thickness of fish. Test the cooking by probing one of the fillets with the blade of a small knife. If the blade goes through easily the fish is cooked. Take care not to overcook the fish.

Serve immediately, spreading a little pesto sauce on top.

SERVING SUGGESTION: Serve with grilled tomatoes, steamed beans and steamed potatoes.

Mediterranean fish in foil

This dish can be varied in many ways. The recipe here has a Mediterranean flavour and uses herbs, but if you want an Asian touch, try using ginger, soy sauce and curry spices. Slice the vegetables finely so that they will cook quickly.

SERVES 1

4 leaves of flat-leaved parsley or 1 small sprig curly parsley

2 slices tomato

freshly ground black pepper

3 basil leaves, shredded

3 mushrooms, sliced

a 150 g (5 oz) fish fillet of your choice

Wash and slice parsley.

Preheat oven to 200°C/400°F.

Cut a strip of foil about 25 cm (about 10 in) square. In the centre, place two slices of tomato, season with a little pepper and on top place half the basil and half the mushroom. Then add parsley and fish fillet and season with more pepper. Lastly, sprinkle with remaining basil and mushroom. Fold foil to seal fish parcels tightly and place in oven to cook for 8 to 10 mins, depending on the thickness of the fish.

SERVING SUGGESTION: Eat as a first course and follow with a dish of vegetables and rice.

Madras fish curry with coriander

This is a Madras-style curry so it is a little hot, but not quite as hot as an Indian would make it. Most firm fish can be used and for this dish at home I use flathead fillets. Don't worry about the long list of ingredients: this delicious dish takes a little longer than a grill, but it is very easy to prepare.

SERVES ABOUT 4

600 g (about 1¼ lb) fish fillets or cutlets

juice of ½ lemon

1 tsp tamarind concentrate (available in Asian grocery shops)

1 cup hot water (from the kettle)

a 1 cm (⅓ in) piece of ginger

3 cloves garlic, peeled

½ cup fresh coriander leaves

1 green chilli, seeds removed

1 tbsp peanut oil

½ brown onion, chopped

1½ tsp ground cummin

1½ tsp ground coriander

2 tsp turmeric

½ tsp chilli powder

freshly ground black pepper

Cut fish into four portions and marinate in lemon juice.

In a bowl dilute tamarind with the hot water.

Peel ginger and blend it to a purée with peeled garlic, coriander leaves and fresh green chilli. Alternatively, chop these ingredients very finely.

Heat oil in a large frying pan or wok. Stir in onion and fry for about 4 mins on low heat. Stir in ground cummin, ground coriander, turmeric, chilli powder and a little pepper and cook for about 2 mins. Add the spicy purée and cook for a further 2 mins. Add diluted tamarind, bring to a simmer and cook for about 10 mins.

Place fish portions in spicy sauce and shake pan, allowing the sauce to coat the top of the fish. Simmer for 3 mins then turn fish over to simmer for another 3 to 5 mins, depending on the thickness of the fillets or cutlets.

When the fish is ready, serve as soon as possible.

SERVING SUGGESTION: Serve with rice and cauliflower.

When baking or pan-frying fish, use a pan just large enough, otherwise the natural juices will burn in the extra space.

Asian baked fish

Ask your fishmonger to gut and scale the fresh fish you select. Fish belonging to the snapper family is always delicious prepared this way. There is a photograph of the dish opposite page 85.

SERVES ABOUT 4

2 tsp honey

1 tsp peanut or polyunsaturated oil

1 small hot chilli, seeded and finely sliced

1 tsp grated ginger

1 tsp lemon juice

½ tsp sesame oil

2 tsp salt-reduced soy sauce

a 1 kg (about 2 lb) whole fish, gutted and scaled

2 spring onions, cut into 2.5 cm (1 in) pieces

In a small bowl thoroughly mix honey, peanut oil, chilli, ginger, lemon juice, sesame oil and soy sauce.

Rinse the inside of the fish and pat fish dry using a clean towel. Make five or six shallow crosscuts about 1 cm (⅓ in) deep on both sides of the fish. This helps the fish cook more evenly.

Preheat oven to 200°C/400°F.

Brush fish all over with marinade. Place fish in a greased oven dish and cook in preheated oven for about 20 mins. Cover fish tail with a small piece of foil during the cooking if it starts browning too much.

Carefully transfer fish with any pan juices to a serving dish and sprinkle with spring onion.

SERVING SUGGESTION: Serve with rice and watercress.

Red emperor stew with vegetables

Prepare this fish stew using any fairly firm, large fish, such as silver trevally, deep-sea trevalla, kingfish or barramundi. This is truly quick cuisine – simple to prepare, quick to cook and sensational to taste.

SERVES ABOUT 4

3 sticks celery

2 medium carrots

1 tsp peanut or polyunsaturated oil

¼ white onion, finely chopped

1 tsp grated ginger

1 cup water

a pinch of saffron

a 500 g (about 1 lb) red emperor fillet, skinned

¼ tsp hot chilli paste

freshly ground black pepper

2 tbsp fresh coriander leaves or 2 tbsp flat-leaved parsley

Wash celery and cut diagonally into bite-size pieces.

Peel carrots, halve lengthwise then cut diagonally into bite-size pieces.

In a large saucepan heat oil and gently stir-fry onion and ginger for 2 mins. Add celery and carrot and stir-fry for about 2 mins without browning. Add water and saffron, cover and cook until vegetables are almost soft.

Cut fillet into bite-size strips. Add to vegetables and cook on high heat for about 3 mins. Turn off heat, cover and leave to rest for 2 mins. Season with chilli paste, a little black pepper and washed coriander leaves.

SERVING SUGGESTION: Serve with Asian noodles.

Spicy scallops with celery

My wife Angie and I love scallops and this is a delicious way to prepare them using a minimum of fat. Scallops are a favourite with fast-food cooks. They must not be cooked for long or they will shrink and lose their tender, moist quality.

SERVES 2

300 g (11 oz) fresh scallops
1 tsp peanut oil
1 tbsp chopped onion
1 cup chopped celery
½ cup water
½ tsp grated ginger
¼ tsp hot chilli paste
freshly ground black pepper
¼ clove garlic, chopped
1 tbsp chopped parsley
a few drops lemon juice

Wash scallops and trim off any rubbery pieces.

Brush a medium saucepan with oil, add onion and celery, and cook for 2 mins on medium heat. Add ½ cup water, bring to boil and cook on high heat until there is about 1 tbsp of liquid left. Add scallops and ginger, cover and steam until the scallops change colour. Stir once or twice very gently – altogether this should take about 2 mins.

Season scallops with chilli paste, a little pepper, chopped garlic, parsley and a few drops of lemon juice. Mix gently and serve.

SERVING SUGGESTION: Serve with crusty wholemeal bread.

Baked whole flounder

Ask your fishmonger to clean and scale the fish you select. If you prepare this dish for several people, remember that flounder is a wide fish and takes up quite a bit of space in the oven. To save time, ask your fishmonger to remove all the fins of the fish. If you do it yourself, use scissors. Again, this is really my idea of good food fast – the freshest fish, a brush with some spices, then into the oven to bake.

SERVES 1

½ tsp paprika
a pinch of cayenne pepper
freshly ground black pepper
½ tsp turmeric
1 tsp olive oil
a 250–300 g (9–11 oz) flounder
1 lemon wedge

Preheat oven to 220°C/450°F.

Mix spices and oil in a small bowl and brush fish on both sides with this preparation. Place fish on an oven sheet and bake in preheated oven for about 5 mins. Using a wide spatula turn fish over and bake for a further 3 mins or until cooked.

Serve immediately with the lemon wedge.

SERVING SUGGESTION: Serve with steamed potatoes and broccoli. Personally, I prefer to eat the fish first then have the vegetables as a second course.

Filo fish parcels

Choose a flathead large enough for two people and ask your fishmonger to fillet and skin it for you. You can, of course, use another type of fish. Handle the filo pastry very gently. With a little practice you will find it quite easy to work with.

SERVES 2

2 skinned flathead fillets, 100–150 g (3½–5 oz) each

freshly ground black pepper

1 tsp curry powder or mixed spices of your choice

a little peanut or polyunsaturated oil

2 sheets of wholemeal filo pastry

Season fish fillets with a little pepper and curry powder.

Preheat oven to 220°C/450°F.

Place two sheets of filo pastry on your work bench and brush with a little oil. Place one fish fillet on each sheet and gently wrap the fish in the pastry, rolling it up completely. Transfer carefully to a baking sheet, tucking the edges of the pastry underneath to seal the parcel well. Brush the top with a little oil and, using the tip of a blade, make two small holes on top of the pastry to allow excess moisture to escape.

Bake in preheated oven for about 12 mins until pastry is crisp and golden brown.

Serve immediately or the moisture of the fish will soften the pastry.

SERVING SUGGESTION: Serve with a mixed salad.

Turkish fish kebabs

Once cooked, fish kebabs should be served immediately, otherwise they lose their moisture and delicate flavour. Ask your fishmonger for a firm fish, such as gurnard, flathead or tuna. The suggested seasoning of paprika and lemon juice is common to Turkish tables. If you prefer an Italian effect use basil and lemon juice, or for a Greek touch try oregano and lemon. Allow 2 hrs for the fish to marinate before cooking, and remember to soak your bamboo sticks for at least 30 mins beforehand to prevent them from burning. Once on the grill, the fish is ready in minutes.

MAKES ABOUT 8 KEBABS

600 g (1¼ lb) firm fish fillets

1½ tbsp olive oil

1 tsp lemon juice

2 tsp finely chopped onion

2 bay leaves broken into pieces

a pinch of salt

freshly ground black pepper

½ tsp paprika

Cut fish into approximately 3 cm (1½ in) cubes and add to a bowl containing olive oil, lemon juice, onion, bay leaves, salt, pepper and paprika. Allow to marinate for about 2 hrs.

Thread fish onto bamboo sticks or skewers and cook on a hot barbecue, turning kebabs over halfway through the cooking. They need about 3 mins on each side and during the cooking they can be brushed with any leftover marinade.

Serve immediately.

SERVING SUGGESTION: Serve with a mixed salad, good bread and rice.

Quicker Chicken, Turkey and Quail

Times certainly change! Only four years ago when *Family Food*, the first cookbook in this series, was published, many people were surprised at the thought of skinning chicken to make a casserole or stew, or when pan-frying a chicken breast. Nowadays, the best-selling chicken cuts from my local poultry shop are skinless and the most popular cut of all is the very lean chicken breast. Poulterers are creative in the variety of cuts they produce from a chicken. Take a chicken thigh, for instance. It comes whole, boneless or diced, and all three are available with or without the skin. Having such a choice gives us the opportunity of buying just what we need, and is very convenient for small households. And, of course, for the busy cook, it saves precious time. We need to remember, though, that portioned chicken has the disadvantage of losing its freshness more rapidly than a whole chicken, so it is preferable to cook it on the day it is purchased, or at least the following day. If you are not sure about the freshness of your meat, smell it. When chicken is off, the smell is rather unpleasant. The smell test is applicable to most meats available from the poulterers, for example turkey, duck, quail and rabbit. Portioned chicken may appear more expensive at first glance but remember there is very little waste.

Perhaps the speediest recipes in this chapter are those for oriental drumsticks and family chicken burgers.

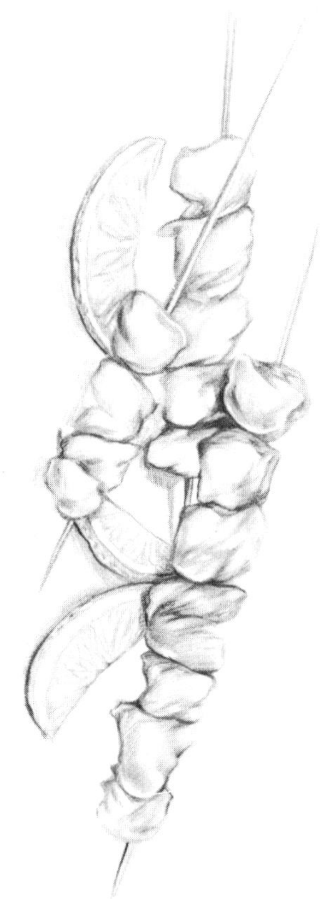

Stir-fried chicken strips cook in minutes.

Aromatic chicken and spinach curry (page 105) is a marvellous one-dish dinner, or you can serve it with traditional dhal (page 69)

Selecting and preparing chicken

Once cooked, a fresh chicken is more flavoursome and has a firmer, juicier texture than a chicken that has been frozen. Choose a strong-looking bird with a plump, meaty breast, robust legs and fairly taut skin. Loose skin usually indicates a lack of freshness. The colour may vary from one breed to another and, depending on what the chicken was fed on, is generally fleshy pink rather than off-white. A free-range chicken costs a bit more but in my opinion usually tastes better and loses less weight during cooking than a battery chicken. Overall, the chicken available in Australia is not as flavoursome as breeds available in some other countries. Food lovers hope these breeds will be introduced to this country.

A 1.2 kg (2 lb 7 oz) chicken is usually sufficient to serve four average-sized adults. At home a chicken weighing 1 kg (about 2 lb) satisfies the appetite of our family, consisting of two adults and two children, and there is usually a little left over for sandwiches the next day. When preparing a dish using chicken pieces, allow per person about 180–200 g (6½–7 oz) with the bone, and about 125–150 g (4–5 oz) without the bone.

Skinning chicken is an easy procedure. With one hand, pull the skin away from the chicken, using the blade of a knife held in the other hand to detach it as you go. If occasionally you wish to leave the skin on a whole chicken, trim off all excess fat and skin at the neck and tail part of the bird. After skinning chicken pieces, such as the thigh, you can also trim a little fat from around the flesh. The fattiest chicken pieces, such as the wing, may be difficult to skin but a little fat can be trimmed off, using a sharp knife. Store your chicken bones in the freezer for preparing a chicken stock at a later date.

The recipes in this chapter illustrate various ways of seasoning and cooking chicken. Some of the quickest (and perhaps the most delicious) ways of serving chicken are also the easiest and healthiest. Avoid overcooking chicken, as people compensate for dried-out chicken by adding more seasoning with salt and more fat than for moist chicken. Go for dishes that require a minimal amount of fat. Deep-fried chicken is best consumed only very occasionally, and be aware that the marinades used to flavour chicken pieces and kebabs in poultry shops may contain high levels of salt, sugar and fat.

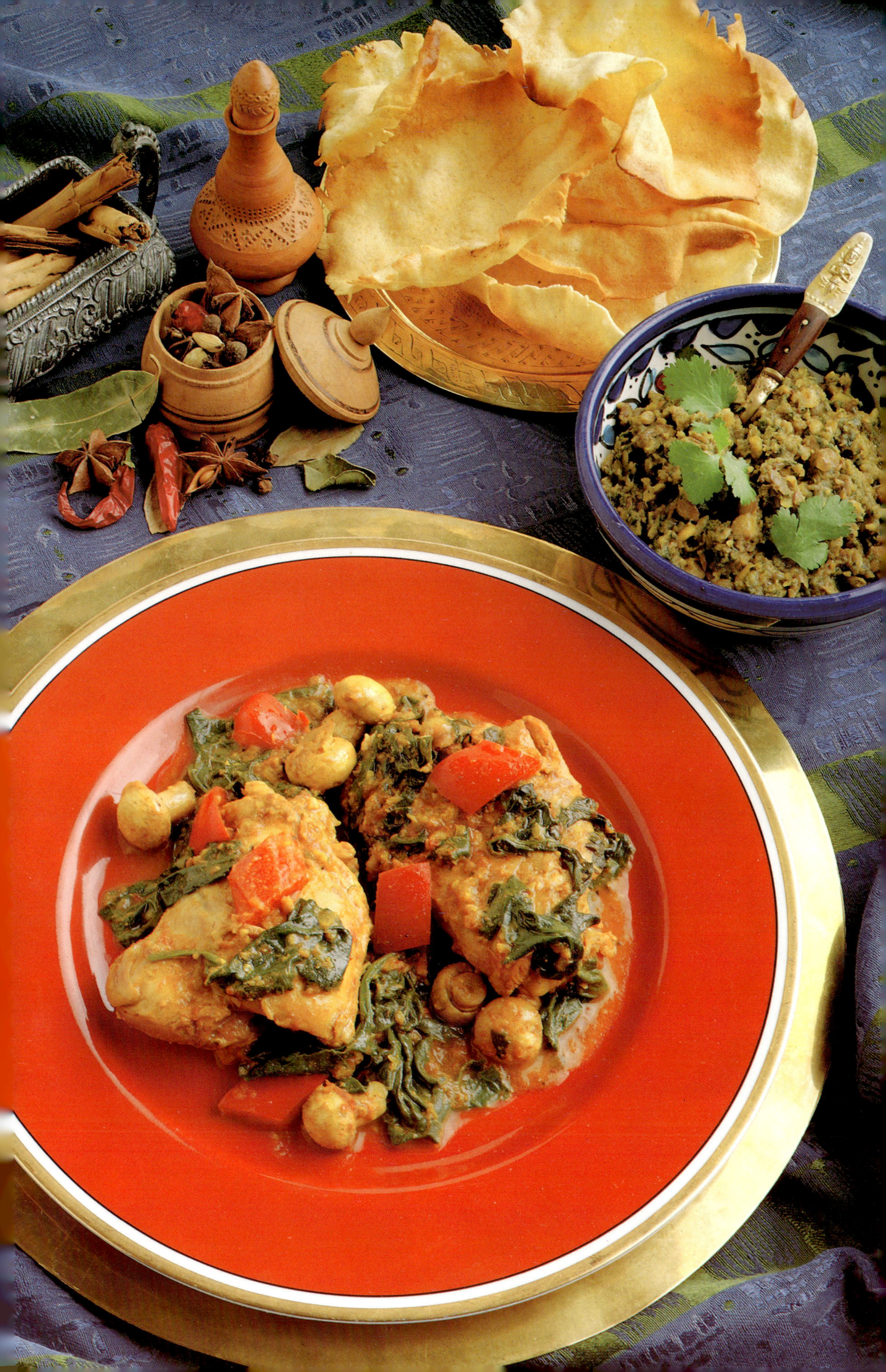

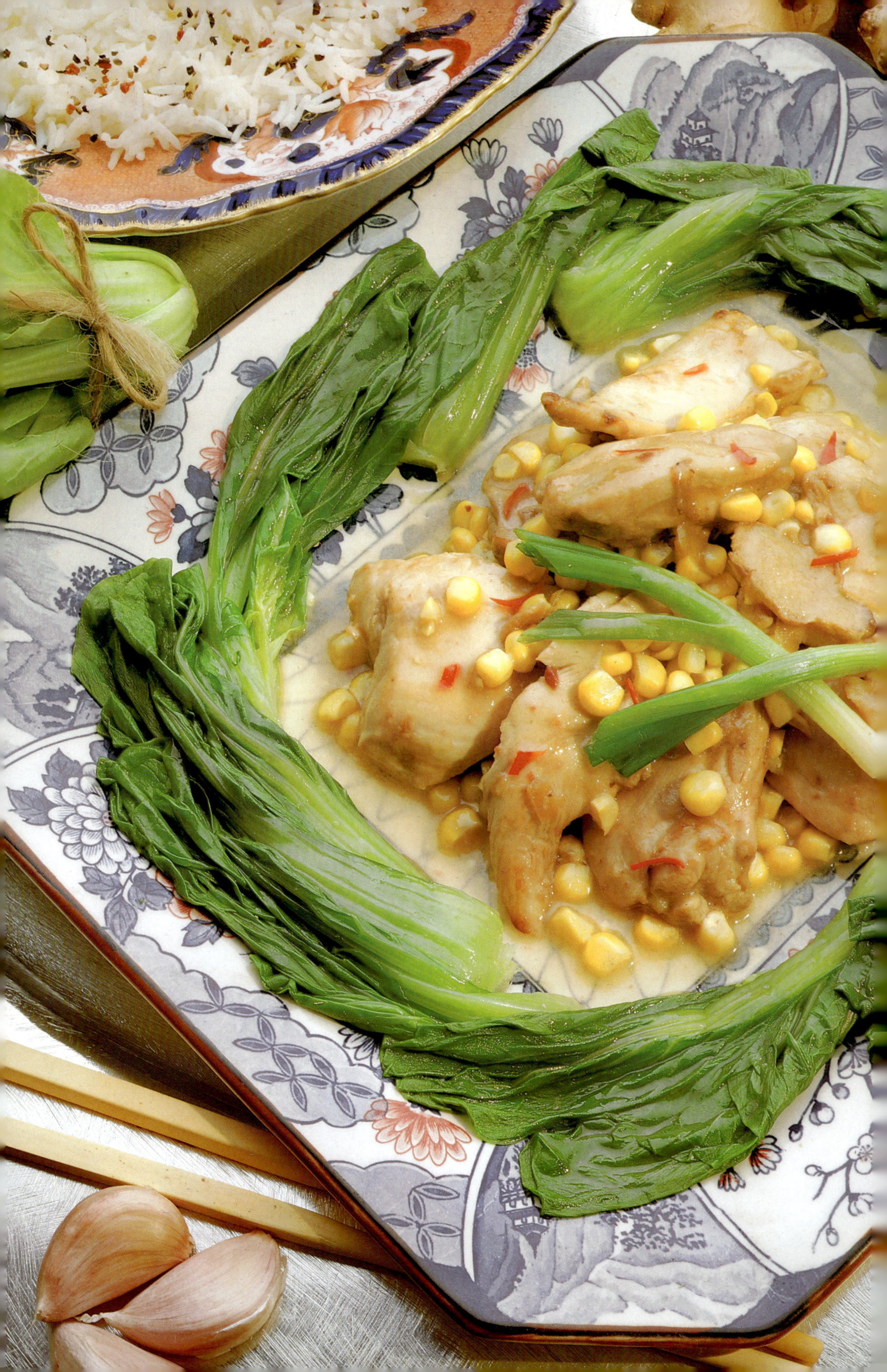

Family chicken burgers

Burgers can be made with all types of lean minced meat and the secret for success is a good seasoning. As you will see in this recipe, your lean meat burgers stay moist if you combine the meat well with a little cold water in a bowl. Minced meat deteriorates rapidly so it is preferable to make burgers on the day of purchase. Make your burgers flat, not fat, to speed the cooking time.

SERVES 4

¼ **brown onion**

500 g (about 1 lb) lean minced chicken

1 tbsp dried breadcrumbs

1 tbsp chopped parsley

1 tbsp bottled or home-made Italian tomato sauce (chapter 7)

3 tbsp water

freshly ground black pepper

a little plain flour

a little olive oil

Peel onion and chop very finely.

In a bowl thoroughly mix onion, minced chicken, breadcrumbs, parsley, tomato sauce, water and a little pepper. This is best done by hand. Divide this mixture into four, and shape four burgers. Coat burgers with a little flour.

Brush a small frying pan with olive oil and cook meat on both sides for about 3 to 4 mins. The chicken meat must be cooked through but not dry.

SERVING SUGGESTION: Serve with wholemeal rolls and salad.

Chicken fillets with a golden sauce

Chicken fillets are the most popular of all chicken cuts and, according to my poulterer, it is because 'they are fast to cook and children like them'. No need for any other reason!

SERVES ABOUT 4

½ **red capsicum**

1 cup pumpkin flesh, cut into cubes

3 tbsp water

a little peanut or polyunsaturated oil

4 chicken fillets

juice of ½ lemon

2 tbsp chopped parsley

1 tbsp grated parmesan cheese

freshly ground black pepper

Wash capsicum and remove seeds. Dice capsicum.

Place diced capsicum and pumpkin cubes in a saucepan with 3 tbsp water, cover and cook until pumpkin is soft. It takes about 5 mins.

Meanwhile, brush a frying pan with a little oil and, when hot, cook chicken fillets on both sides on medium heat. It takes about 10 mins.

Meanwhile, blend pumpkin and capsicum with their cooking liquid to a smooth sauce, adding a little water if necessary.

When the chicken is cooked, add lemon juice to pan and shake pan lightly before adding the vegetable sauce. Reheat and serve chicken sprinkled with parsley and cheese and seasoned with a little pepper.

◁
Chicken and Chinese bok choy stir-fried in a wok for a fast meal without fuss (page 104)

Spicy chicken kebabs

When preparing kebabs you can be creative, using spices and seasonings according to your mood. Soak bamboo sticks in water for at least 30 mins before use to prevent the wood from burning. The dish can be cooked on the barbecue, in a pan, under the grill or in the oven.

MAKES ABOUT 8 KEBABS

400 g (14 oz) deboned chicken meat (fillet or thigh)

juice of ½ lemon

¼ tsp hot chilli paste

1 tsp fennel seeds or cummin seeds

½ tsp paprika

freshly ground black pepper

½–1 tbsp peanut oil

16 small mushrooms

1 small red capsicum

4 small zucchini

Skin chicken and cut into regular bite-size pieces. In a mixing bowl toss chicken with lemon juice, chilli, fennel seeds, paprika, a little pepper and oil.

Prepare vegetables by cutting them into regular pieces no bigger than the chicken, and mix them well with chicken. Thread vegetables and chicken onto sticks, alternating as you go to make kebabs as attractive as possible. Refrigerate until required.

Place kebabs under a medium grill not too close to the flame and cook for about 5 mins on each side. Alternatively, cook on a clean, hot barbecue, in a frying pan brushed with oil, or on a rack in a hot oven.

SERVING SUGGESTION: Serve with rice or a mixed salad, or remove from sticks and enjoy in a wholemeal roll or in pita bread.

Oriental drumsticks

We have cooked this dish many times at home and our children love it. For best results, put the drumsticks on a rack to allow the oven heat to circulate around the meat and cook it evenly. If preparing this dish for adults you may wish to add ¼ tsp of chilli and 1 tsp of grated ginger. The dish is seen in our photograph opposite page 52.

SERVES 4

1 tsp honey

1 tsp salt-reduced soy sauce

juice of ½ lemon

½ clove garlic, finely chopped

3 drops sesame oil

freshly ground black pepper

4 chicken drumsticks

Preheat oven to 180°C/350°F.

In a small bowl mix together honey, soy sauce, lemon juice, garlic, sesame oil and a little pepper.

Skin drumsticks and coat with the marinade preparation. Place drumsticks on a rack, turning them over halfway through the cooking, and cook for about 30 mins or until chicken is cooked.

SERVING SUGGESTION: Serve with stir-fried green vegetables and Asian noodles.

Island chicken with vegetables

This is a delicately spiced chicken dish with a strong contrast of colour and texture. Don't be put off by the long list of ingredients. This dish is quite easy to make, and with some fast-cooking Asian noodles you will have an exotic and nutritious meal.

SERVES 4

600 g (1¼ lb) small skinless chicken pieces on the bone

1 tbsp plain flour

2 zucchini

1 red capsicum

1 small brown onion

½–1 tbsp peanut oil

½ tsp turmeric

½ tsp curry powder

1 cup water

1 tbsp desiccated coconut

1 tbsp raw peanuts

freshly ground black pepper

a few fresh coriander leaves

Coat chicken pieces with flour.

Wash and slice zucchini. Halve, seed, wash and finely slice capsicum.

Peel onion and slice finely.

Heat oil in a large saucepan, and brown chicken pieces for a few minutes. Transfer chicken to a plate. Add onion to pan and gently cook for 2 mins before adding zucchini, capsicum, turmeric and curry powder. Stir for about 2 mins to prevent burning. Add water and chicken pieces, stir again and bring to boil. Reduce to a simmer, cover and cook for 25 mins or until chicken is cooked.

Add coconut and peanuts, season with a little pepper, stir gently and cook uncovered for a further 5 mins. Sprinkle with coriander leaves and serve.

SERVING SUGGESTION: Serve with Asian noodles or brown rice.

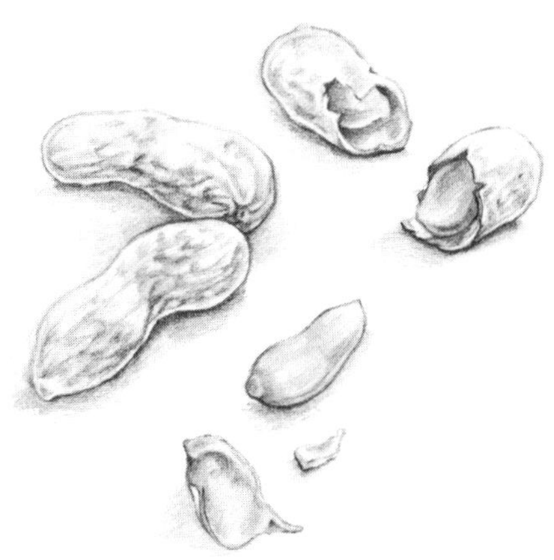

Chinese stir-fry chicken with bok choy

It is easy to become familiar with the Chinese stir-frying technique, a vital one for the busy cook. The secret is to practise with simple dishes like this one. Ordinary cabbage (one-quarter) can replace the bok choy. The dish is shown in the photograph opposite page 101.

SERVES 4

400 g (14 oz) deboned chicken meat (fillet or thigh)

2 tsp dry sherry

1 tbsp salt-reduced soy sauce

2 tsp cornflour

2–4 bok choy (a type of Chinese cabbage), depending on size

2 cobs of corn or a 400 g (14 oz) can corn kernels (no added salt), drained

½ brown onion

1 clove garlic

1 tbsp peanut oil

2 thin slices ginger

1 cup water

1 tbsp cold water

1 small hot chilli, finely sliced and seeded (optional)

2 spring onions, cut diagonally into bite-size pieces

Remove skin of chicken and trim off all the fat. Cut chicken into bite-size pieces. In a bowl mix chicken pieces with sherry, half the soy sauce and half the cornflour.

Bring a large saucepan of water to boil.

Cut bok choy in half lengthwise and cut each half into three lengthwise. Wash and cook in boiling water for 2 mins then drain.

Using a short, sharp knife, remove corn kernels from cobs, or drain a can of corn kernels.

Peel and dice brown onion and peel and crush garlic.

Heat wok for a few seconds then heat oil in hot wok. Add onion, garlic and ginger and stir-fry for a few seconds. Add chicken pieces and stir-fry for a few minutes until chicken is browned. Transfer chicken to a plate. Pour 1 cup water into wok, bring to boil and add corn and bok choy. Return to boil, cover and cook for about 5 mins until bok choy is cooked but still crunchy.

In a small bowl combine remaining cornflour with 1 tbsp cold water and stir into wok. Add chicken pieces, remaining soy sauce and chilli. Stir well and reheat on low heat for 3 to 4 mins.

If you wish, remove garlic and ginger, before serving sprinkled with spring onion.

Chicken and spinach curry

This is a marvellous one-dish dinner – easy to prepare for a large number of people, especially if you use a wok. The curry appears in our photograph opposite page 100.

SERVES 4

1 bunch spinach

4 chicken thighs, skinned

½ brown onion

a 2 cm (¾ in) piece of ginger

2 cloves garlic

2 tomatoes

100 g (3½ oz) small button mushrooms

1 tbsp peanut oil

½ tsp fennel seeds

2 tsp curry powder

½ tsp hot chilli paste (optional)

Detach spinach leaves from stalks and wash leaves two or three times in a large quantity of cold water.

Peel onion, ginger and garlic and blend together to a fine purée. Alternatively, chop them finely.

Halve tomatoes, squeeze out seeds and chop tomato finely. Wash mushrooms.

Heat wok for a few seconds. Then heat oil in wok, add fennel seeds and puréed onion, ginger and garlic, and cook on medium heat without browning for 3 or 4 mins. Add curry powder and stir well for about 30 secs before adding tomato.

Bring to boil, add chicken thighs and whole mushrooms, cover wok and cook for 20 mins. Stir well then place spinach leaves on top. Cover wok and cook until spinach has softened – it takes only a few minutes. Remove lid and stir chicken with spinach. Season with chilli paste and serve.

SERVING SUGGESTION: Serve with wholegrain rice and Indian breads.

Malaysian chicken satay

This is the dish that our children often ask for after enjoying satays in a local Malaysian restaurant. The seasoning can be adapted to your taste. Soak 20 small bamboo sticks in cold water for at least 30 mins before cooking to prevent them from burning.

SERVES 4

4 chicken fillets or deboned thighs

juice of ¼ lemon

1 tsp salt-reduced soy sauce

1 tsp honey

½ tsp turmeric

¼ tsp curry powder

¼ tsp (or less) hot chilli paste

1 tsp peanut oil

freshly ground black pepper

1 extra tsp peanut oil, if pan-frying

4 lemon wedges

Skin chicken fillets and cut in half horizontally. Then cut each piece into small strips about 5 cm (2 in) long and ½ cm (¼ in) thick.

In a medium bowl, mix lemon juice, soy sauce, honey, turmeric, curry powder, chilli paste, oil and a little pepper. Toss chicken in this marinade, and refrigerate for at least 30 mins. This can be done in the morning for a speedy meal in the evening.

Thread meat lengthwise onto kebabs and cook under grill. Alternatively, cook in a frying pan brushed with a little oil, on a barbecue or in a hot oven on a rack. The satays will take only a few minutes to cook, and they are much tastier moist than overcooked and dry.

Serve with lemon wedges or with satay sauce.

SERVING SUGGESTION: Serve with rice and a green vegetable.

Mon coq au vin

Chicken cooked in wine is a classic of French cooking and every French region has its own version. Coq au vin requires a little more time than many people can spare for a mid-week meal, but it is marvellous for a special dinner and not at all hard to make.

SERVES 4

1 carrot

1 onion

1 stick celery

12 small mushrooms

1 slice lean bacon

4 large chicken thighs

a little plain flour

a little polyunsaturated oil

1 tbsp brandy

¾ cup red wine

**½ cup chicken stock
(chapter 7)**

**½ cup bottled or home-
made Italian tomato sauce
(chapter 7)**

½ bay leaf

freshly ground black pepper

about 1 cup shelled peas

1 tbsp chopped parsley

Peel carrot, onion and celery, and dice finely. Wash mushrooms.

Cut bacon into small strips.

Skin chicken thighs and coat with a little flour.

Heat two medium saucepans brushed with a little oil. In one of them cook carrot, onion and celery on medium heat. In the second saucepan fry bacon for 2 mins. Transfer bacon to a bowl, and to the same saucepan add chicken thighs and brown them. Transfer chicken to the saucepan containing the vegetables, and in the empty saucepan cook mushrooms on high heat for about 5 mins or until cooked. Transfer mushrooms to bowl with bacon.

Add brandy to empty saucepan and bring to boil. Add wine and stock, and return to boil before adding tomato sauce. Pour this liquid over chicken and stir well, adding bay leaf and seasoning with a little pepper. Bring to a simmer, cover and cook for 25 mins.

Add peas, stir and cook uncovered for a further 10 mins. Add bacon, mushrooms and chopped parsley, stir through to reheat and serve.

Chicken pancakes with herbs

This dish is ideally suited to occasions such as having one or two guests for an informal light lunch. Serve with a mixed salad and perhaps follow with a fresh fruit salad. Prepare your pancake batter first, then leave for at least 30 mins while you make the filling. Pancakes can be made in advance (for example, the night before) and reheated, which saves last-minute cooking.

MAKES 4–6 PANCAKES

3 tbsp plain white flour

4 tbsp plain wholemeal flour

1 egg

1 cup low-fat milk

a pinch of salt

a pinch of cayenne pepper

300 g (11 oz) deboned chicken meat (fillet or thigh)

2 tsp olive oil

12 small mushrooms, sliced

½ clove garlic, finely chopped

3 tbsp bottled or home-made Italian tomato sauce (chapter 7)

1 tbsp chopped parsley

1 tbsp chopped basil

freshly ground black pepper

1 tsp polyunsaturated margarine or butter

Place both types of flour in a bowl and make a hollow in the centre. Into the hollow pour the egg, half of the milk, salt and cayenne pepper. Using a whisk, first mix egg and milk together then gradually incorporate flour, slowly adding the rest of the milk to form a smooth mixture. Refrigerate for at least 30 mins.

Skin chicken and cut into bite-size pieces.

In a small saucepan, heat half olive oil, add sliced mushrooms and cook on high heat for 30 secs. Add chicken pieces and garlic, and cook for a further 3 mins before adding tomato sauce, parsley and half of the basil. Season with a little pepper and put aside.

Add remaining basil to pancake batter.

Brush pancake pan with remaining olive oil, and margarine, and when the margarine has melted, pour into pancake batter. Return pan to heat and, using a ladle, thinly cover bottom of pan with mixture. Twirl pan smoothly to form a thin, even pancake.

When upper half of pancake starts to dry, turn pancake over, using a wide spatula. After browning second side, remove pancake and start cooking another immediately without adding any more margarine or oil to pan.

Spoon about 2 tbsp chicken preparation onto each pancake and roll pancakes up neatly. Place on a serving dish and reheat a little in a low oven before serving.

Paella with chicken and prawns

Paella is a traditional rice dish garnished with vegetables, chicken and shellfish, which is easy to prepare. An added bonus for busy cooks and their families — it only requires one saucepan, so even cleaning up is easy.

SERVES ABOUT 4

1 small brown onion

1 clove garlic

1 red capsicum

1 tomato

1 tbsp olive oil

4 small chicken thighs, skinned

1 cup shelled peas

1 cup long-grain brown rice

3 cups cold water

2 pinches of saffron

freshly ground black pepper

8–12 green prawns

Peel and finely slice onion.

Peel and crush garlic.

Halve, seed and wash capsicum.

Wash and dice tomato.

Heat oil in a heavy saucepan and brown chicken pieces. Add onion and garlic, stir-fry for 1 min then add capsicum, tomato, peas, rice and water. Bring to boil and season with saffron and a little pepper. Stir gently, cover and simmer for 30 mins.

After this time, add prawns, stir gently, cover and cook for a further 5 mins. Add a little extra water towards the end of cooking if necessary.

SERVING SUGGESTION: Serve in a large serving dish from the centre of the table, perhaps accompanied by a green salad.

Baked poussin Mexican-style

A poussin is a young chicken that is exceptionally tender, and ideal for sharing between two people when served with vegetables. As the poussin is very small, it will only take about 25 mins to cook — a very quick roast I'm sure you'll agree.

SERVES 2

2 tbsp bottled or home-made Italian tomato sauce (chapter 7)

2 tsp olive oil

½ tsp cummin

½ tsp hot chilli paste

¼ tsp coriander powder

freshly ground black pepper

1 poussin

¼ lemon

In a small bowl thoroughly mix tomato sauce, half of the olive oil, cummin, chilli paste, coriander and a little pepper.

Preheat oven to 180°C/350°F.

Using poultry scissors or a large knife or cleaver, halve poussin and remove neck, and liver and lungs from inside the carcass if necessary. Remove skin of the bird.

Brush a small roasting tray with remaining oil. Place poussin in tray and spread the seasoned tomato paste over the bird. Bake in preheated oven for 15 mins then turn bird over and bake for a further 10 mins.

Squeeze a few drops of lemon juice over poussin before serving.

SERVING SUGGESTION: Serve with brown rice and steamed beans.

Greek barbecued quails

Quails are very tasty and a delight for those who enjoy sucking bones. You can prepare the seasoning and the quails the day before if you wish. The quails can be barbecued or baked on a rack in a hot oven. The oregano may be replaced with basil or parsley.

SERVES 4

4 quails
1 tbsp olive oil
1 tsp oregano
freshly ground black pepper
a pinch of salt
4 lemon wedges

Using poultry scissors or a large knife or cleaver, cut quails in half.

In a small bowl mix olive oil with oregano, a little pepper and salt. Brush quails all over with this preparation and leave to marinate in the refrigerator for at least a few hours.

Cook quails on a hot, clean barbecue and serve with lemon wedges.

SERVING SUGGESTION: Serve with a variety of salads.

Florentine turkey breast

Until recently turkey was usually reserved for sharing with the family at Christmas time. But now in many specialist shops various cuts of turkey, such as the legs, steaks from the breast meat, and whole breasts are available. These smaller portions make them ideal for people who enjoy something a little different, but who have limited time. This pot-roasted turkey breast is a superb dish for a special occasion.

SERVES 4

1 bunch spinach
3 tbsp water
12 mushrooms
a pinch of nutmeg
freshly ground black pepper
a 600 g (1¼ lb) turkey breast
1 carrot
½ brown onion
1 stick celery
½–1 tbsp olive oil
1 sprig lemon thyme, chopped

Detach spinach leaves from stalks and wash them two or three times in a large quantity of cold water.

Place spinach in a large saucepan with 2 tbsp of the water, cover and cook until spinach is soft – it takes only a few minutes. Transfer spinach to a bowl.

Wash and slice mushrooms and cook on high heat in a saucepan with 1 tbsp water for a few minutes. Transfer mushroom to bowl with spinach, and season with nutmeg and a little pepper. Stir well.

Make a small incision in the turkey breast to make a pocket, but don't slit right through. Spoon about 4 tbsp of the vegetable preparation into the pocket. Peel and finely dice carrot, onion and celery.

Heat oil in a stove-top casserole dish and lightly brown turkey breast on each side for a few minutes. Place chopped carrot, onion, celery and thyme around turkey, cover and cook on low heat for 10 mins. Stir vegetables well, turn turkey breast over and cook, covered, for another 5 mins.

Add remaining spinach and mushroom to turkey and vegetables and gently reheat for 5 mins.

Carve turkey into 4 pieces, season with more freshly ground black pepper and serve on top of vegetables.

Lean Meat Meals

My cooking activities take me to places all over Australia. It is a big, beautiful country whether you visit a tropical fruit farm in northern Queensland or an onion field in Tasmania, and with its wonderful variety it is a delight to the eye.

Surprisingly (for me), a butcher in Darwin displays much the same meat as a butcher thousands of kilometres away in Hobart, and in my travels most butchers I have chatted with report that lamb chops, minced meat, sausages and steak are the most popular cuts of meat in this country. In rural areas, an Australian butcher is likely to be the sole choice one has, but in the cities there is a greater choice of butchers. Asian butchers specialise in pork, which is more favoured in Asian cooking than beef and lamb. Asian butchers trim their meat very well, and it is worthwhile visiting one just to see what I mean. Continental butchers have varied offerings, depending on what country the butcher originates from. Some specialise in veal, others in pork and smallgoods. Whenever I need flavoursome veal, I am usually best satisfied by making my purchase from a continental butcher.

Nonetheless, most butchers offer good-quality meat and it is a wise idea to develop a friendly relationship with one or several butchers in your neighbourhood. When you require a particular cut, tell your butcher what you need it for, and place an advance order if you want something special like roast veal or a boned leg of lamb.

Eating meat

People who do not cook usually eat whatever they are served, so it is up to the cook to provide a well-balanced meal. For some people it has been routine to eat large quantities of fatty meat that are incompatible with long-lasting good health, especially if this food habit has been associated with little variety in the diet. Certainly, meat is an excellent source of protein, iron, minerals and B vitamins. However, because it also contains fat and is often cooked in conjunction with fat, it is recommended that we buy lean cuts of meat, trim meat of all visible fat, and eat moderate portions. It is further suggested that about 125–150 g (4–5 oz) of trimmed meat per day, roughly equivalent to two chops or a small piece of steak, constitutes an adequate adult portion. Ultimately, it is wise to vary the type and cuts of meat we eat and to include fish and meatless meals in our diet. Remember that lean meat is not a 'bad' food – it is the saturated fat often associated with meat that is detrimental to health. In reducing our meat intake the important point is not to replace it with other fatty foods such as pastries (vegetable pies or quiches), high-fat, cheesy dishes (pasta and pizza with lots of extra cheese) or fried vegetable foods (chips or spring rolls).

Choosing meat

Choosing meat confidently calls for some experience. On arriving at a butcher shop, I first of all take a good look at the window display. Sometimes the display gives me an idea for a new dish or a desire to cook something I have not tried for a long time. If visiting a butcher for the first time, I try to assess the overall quality of the meat. A good butcher displays the meat neatly and in interesting ways. The chops and steak are well trimmed of excess fat and gristle and are evenly sliced. A good cut of meat has a firm texture and the colour varies according to the age of the meat – paler meat usually indicates a younger animal.

It is always encouraging when a butcher cuts or slices a piece of meat in front of you as you buy it, as you can see exactly what you are buying. It is no surprise that well-chosen, well-trimmed meat costs a little more than poor-quality meat with which there is wastage. A good butcher provides all-round service, giving customers information and answering queries about ways to cook the meat that has been purchased.

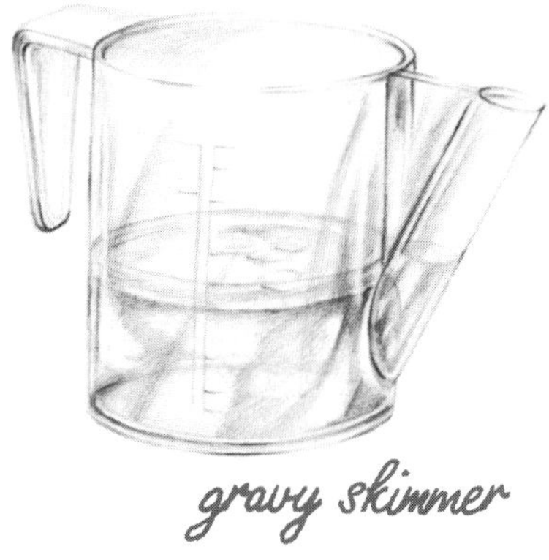

Avoid moving meat constantly in the pan. It slows the cooking process.

Cooking meat

It seems that for the less experienced cook, the most difficult thing to learn about meat is knowing when it is cooked. With steak, chops and hamburgers you need to learn to assess the degree of cooking by touch, that is, by putting a little pressure on the meat with your finger (I use my index finger). Meat is rare when it is brown on top but very soft to the touch. The centre of the meat is, of course, still raw. Meat is medium rare when it is brown on top and offers only a little resistance when touched. In this case, it is pinkish-red in the centre. It is medium when it offers more resistance to the touch but is not quite firm. The centre is still moist and pink. Well-done meat is no longer flexible to the touch, but it is not completely dry and still has a little moisture remaining in the centre. When meat feels hard and dry and there is no moisture remaining inside, it is overdone. This stage should definitely be avoided! The first time you try this technique you may find it hard to judge what is happening. However, after a few attempts, your sense of touch and your concentration will become well tuned and your meat meals will be more delicious.

A meat thermometer helps you cook your roast to the desired degree. It has a spike which is inserted into the centre of the roast towards the end of the cooking. As the roast cooks, the pointer on the dial indicates the temperature at the centre of the meat and tells you if the meat is rare, medium or well done. Meat in a casserole or stew is cooked when it is tender and can be easily chewed. The best way to judge is to taste it, but watch out! It can be hot.

Any meat, whether for grilling, stewing or roasting, cooks better if it has been well trimmed of fat, gristle and skin. A boning knife, sometimes called a butcher's knife, is the most efficient and comfortable knife to use when trimming and deboning meat.

Some of the dishes in this chapter require the meat to be marinated. If you are short of time at the end of the day this may be done in the morning or even the night before. The tender, marinated meat cooks very quickly.

I also include some stir-fry recipes. This is an important technique for the busy cook. Cooking time is very short once you are familiar with it. You will also find some special roasts. These are all, like the classic osso buco, easy and swift to prepare, though the cooking time may be longer. With these recipes I often make double the quantity for a fast and flavoursome dinner on another evening.

Tandoori loin of lamb

To prepare the meat, ask your butcher to debone a rack of lamb having three or four chops, or do it yourself. All fat and skin must be removed so that your loin is very lean. As an alternative, ask your butcher for some lamb or mutton backstrap – about 150 g (5 oz) of meat per person. The meat needs to marinate for at least 1 hr but the result is really tender spicy lamb. I sometimes make the marinade the night before and it only takes me 15 mins to finish the dish.

SERVES ABOUT 4

2 tsp low-fat natural yoghurt

1 tsp grated ginger

¼ tsp freshly ground black pepper

½ tsp paprika

½ tsp cummin seeds

1 tsp curry powder

¼ tsp chilli powder

1 tsp peanut or polyunsaturated oil

½ tsp lemon juice

4 pieces deboned loin of lamb about 10 cm (4 in) long

In a small bowl thoroughly mix yoghurt, ginger, pepper, paprika, cummin seeds, curry powder, chilli powder, oil and lemon juice. Rub all sides of loin of lamb with this spicy preparation and leave to marinate in a cool place for 1 to 4 hrs.

Preheat oven to 250°C/500°F.

Cook loin in a hot, preheated oven on an oven rack resting in an oven dish for about 15 mins. Turn loin over two-thirds of the way through the cooking. To help save time with the washing up later, place a sheet of foil under your oven rack.

SERVING SUGGESTION: Serve with rice or Asian noodles and steamed green vegetables.

Pork chops with apple and onion sauce

Just thinking of this dish reminds me of my childhood. Pork is the meat most often eaten in France, and at home we ate pork chops much more frequently than we ate lamb chops. Avoid overcooking pork, which tends to become dry when overdone.

SERVES 2

1 Granny Smith apple

2 tbsp water

2 pork chops

a little polyunsaturated or peanut oil

½ brown onion, sliced

freshly ground black pepper

Peel, quarter and core apple. Place in a small saucepan with the water, cover and cook until apple is soft.

Trim pork chops of all visible fat. Brush a frying pan with a little oil and on medium heat fry chops on both sides until almost cooked. Remove chops from pan, place on a dish and keep warm in the oven (at 100°C/ 210°F).

Add sliced onion to pan and cook until soft. Then add cooked apple to pan, stir well, season with a little pepper and reheat briefly.

Remove chops from oven. If there is any liquid in the dish, add it to the apple sauce then spoon sauce over chops and serve.

SERVING SUGGESTION: Serve with green vegetables.

Pan-fried lamb chops with basil

Here is a very quick and simple dish of lamb chops with a difference, a dish that the tang of the herbs and lemon transforms into a delightful meal.

SERVES 2

4 loin lamb chops

a little olive oil

½ small clove garlic, chopped

1 tsp chopped parsley

1 tsp finely sliced basil

¼ lemon

freshly ground black pepper

Trim chops of all visible fat.

Brush a frying pan with a little olive oil and on medium heat cook chops on both sides until almost done. Turn off heat. Drain as much fat as possible from frying pan and, leaving chops in pan, cover with a lid or foil and leave chops to rest for 1 min.

Return pan to high heat, stir in garlic, parsley and basil and stir well before squeezing a few drops of lemon juice over chops. Season with a little pepper and serve.

SERVING SUGGESTION: Serve with cauliflower and steamed potatoes.

Veal chops with gremolata

Meat on the bone usually has more flavour than boneless cuts. Veal is a sweet meat, low in fat, and you will find that knowing how to prepare a few veal dishes is a good addition to your cooking repertoire. Gremolata is a classic Italian seasoning of chopped parsley, garlic and grated orange or lemon rind. You will be surprised at how flavoursome this easily prepared dish is.

SERVES 4

2 tomatoes

4 veal chops

a little plain flour

a little olive oil

2 tbsp dry white wine or water

1 tbsp chopped parsley

1 clove garlic, finely chopped

1 tbsp finely grated orange rind

freshly ground black pepper

Halve tomatoes and, after squeezing out the seeds by hand, dice the flesh finely.

Coat chops with a little plain flour.

Brush a frying pan with a little olive oil. When oil is hot cook chops for a few minutes on both sides. Remove chops from pan and keep warm on a serving dish or plate covered with foil or a lid.

Add white wine and tomato to pan and bring to boil for 1 min before stirring in parsley, garlic and orange rind. Season with a little pepper and spoon this sauce over chops.

If you think the chops are not hot enough, reheat them with the sauce in the pan for 1 or 2 mins before serving.

SERVING SUGGESTION: Serve with pasta and steamed broccoli.

Fiery beef kebabs

For meat kebabs to be tender, the fat and gristle on the meat must be trimmed before it is skewered. Try choosing a spicy seasoning of your own but if you lack confidence, try mine and adapt it to your taste next time you make the dish. If using bamboo sticks, to prevent them from burning, soak in cold water for 30 mins before cooking.

MAKES ABOUT 8
KEBABS

600 g (1¼ lb) rump steak, sliced 3 cm (1½ in) thick

1 tsp hot mustard

1 tsp paprika

¼ tsp hot chilli paste

1 tsp ground cummin

1 tsp peanut or polyunsaturated oil

freshly ground black pepper

Trim meat of all fat and gristle and cut into approximately 3 cm (1½ in) cubes.

In a large bowl mix mustard, paprika, hot chilli paste, cummin, oil and pepper. Mix beef cubes with this seasoning and leave to marinate for at least 1 hr, or you can do this in the morning for the evening meal.

Thread meat onto sticks and cook on a barbecue or under a medium grill, turning them halfway through the cooking. Cooking time is 6 to 8 mins in all.

SERVING SUGGESTION: Serve with ratatouille and pasta.

Hungarian beef with paprika

In this stroganoff-style beef dish, I have replaced the cream traditionally used with fresh low-fat soft cheese that has a milk-fat content of less than 8 per cent. The dish is very quickly prepared but do take care not to overcook the meat or it will be dry.

SERVES 2

200 g (7 oz) beef fillet or rump steak

8 medium mushrooms

1 tsp peanut oil

½ small onion, finely chopped

2 tbsp dry white wine

2 tsp ground paprika

freshly ground black pepper

2 tbsp quark (fresh low-fat soft cheese with a milk-fat content of less than 8 per cent)

a few drops lemon juice

1 tbsp chopped parsley

Trim all visible fat from beef. Cut beef into 1 cm (⅓ in) thick slices then into ½ cm (¼ in) thick strips.

Briefly wash mushrooms and slice them.

Brush a frying pan with oil and, when hot, stir-fry beef on high heat for a few seconds until it changes colour. Transfer beef to a bowl.

Add chopped onion to frying pan and on low heat fry for 1 min. Add mushroom, increase heat and stir-fry until mushroom starts to soften. Add wine and bring to boil.

Stir paprika and a little pepper in bowl with beef.

Stir cheese, in pieces, with mushroom and allow cheese to melt but don't boil. Stir in beef and reheat a little.

Squeeze a few drops of lemon juice into pan and add chopped parsley.

Serve immediately.

SERVING SUGGESTION: Serve with pasta or noodles and steamed green vegetables.

Spicy veal osso buco with spinach

This is a truly rustic dish and a good one to enjoy with friends. If rushed, I cook this dish in a pressure cooker as it takes about half the normal time.

SERVES 4

1 small onion

1 small carrot

2 tomatoes

a little plain flour

1 tbsp peanut oil

4 slices shin of veal or beef, about 150 g (5 oz) each

¼ tsp fennel seeds

¼ tsp cummin seeds

½ cup dry white wine

1 cup water

freshly ground black pepper

a large pinch of saffron

1 bunch spinach

Peel and chop onion. Peel and finely dice carrot.

Trim tomatoes and blend to a fine purée.

Coat pieces of veal with flour.

Heat oil in a heavy casserole dish and, on medium heat, brown veal for about 2 mins on each side. Add onion, carrot, fennel and cummin seeds, stir and cook for 2 mins. Add white wine, stir again and add tomato, water, a little pepper and saffron. Bring to a simmer, cover and cook on low heat for about 1½ hrs or until veal meat can be easily detached from the bone.

Detach spinach leaves from stems and wash several times in a large quantity of cold water. Place spinach in casserole without mixing it in, cover pan and cook for a few minutes until spinach is soft. Then gently mix spinach with veal and serve.

SERVING SUGGESTION: Serve with boiled, steamed or microwaved potatoes.

Chinese beef with French beans

Our children love this stir-fry, and my wife Angie and I find it very fast.

SERVES ABOUT 4

300 g (11 oz) rump steak

1 tbsp salt-reduced soy sauce

1 tbsp dry sherry

1 tsp cornflour

400 g (14 oz) French beans

200 g (7 oz) Asian noodles

1 tbsp peanut or polyunsaturated oil

½ clove garlic, crushed

1 thin slice ginger

¼ cup water

1 tsp hot chilli paste

▷

Tender beef fillet, stuffed with silver beet and slivered mushrooms – creative cuisine for the healthy gourmet (page 120)

Trim beef of all fat and cut into bite-size strips. In a bowl mix beef with soy sauce, sherry and cornflour.

Bring a large saucepan of water and a medium saucepan of water to the boil. Wash, top and tail beans. Place beans in boiling water for 1 min. Drain beans.

In the medium saucepan cook noodles in boiling water, following packet instructions.

Heat two-thirds of the oil in a wok. Add garlic, slice of ginger and beef and stir-fry until meat has browned. Transfer meat to a plate and discard ginger.

Pour remaining oil into wok and stir-fry beans for about 15 secs before pouring ¼ cup water down the wok.

Stir well, cover and cook until beans are tender but still crunchy. Then add beef, noodles and chilli paste, or serve chilli paste separately if you wish; stir well to reheat and serve.

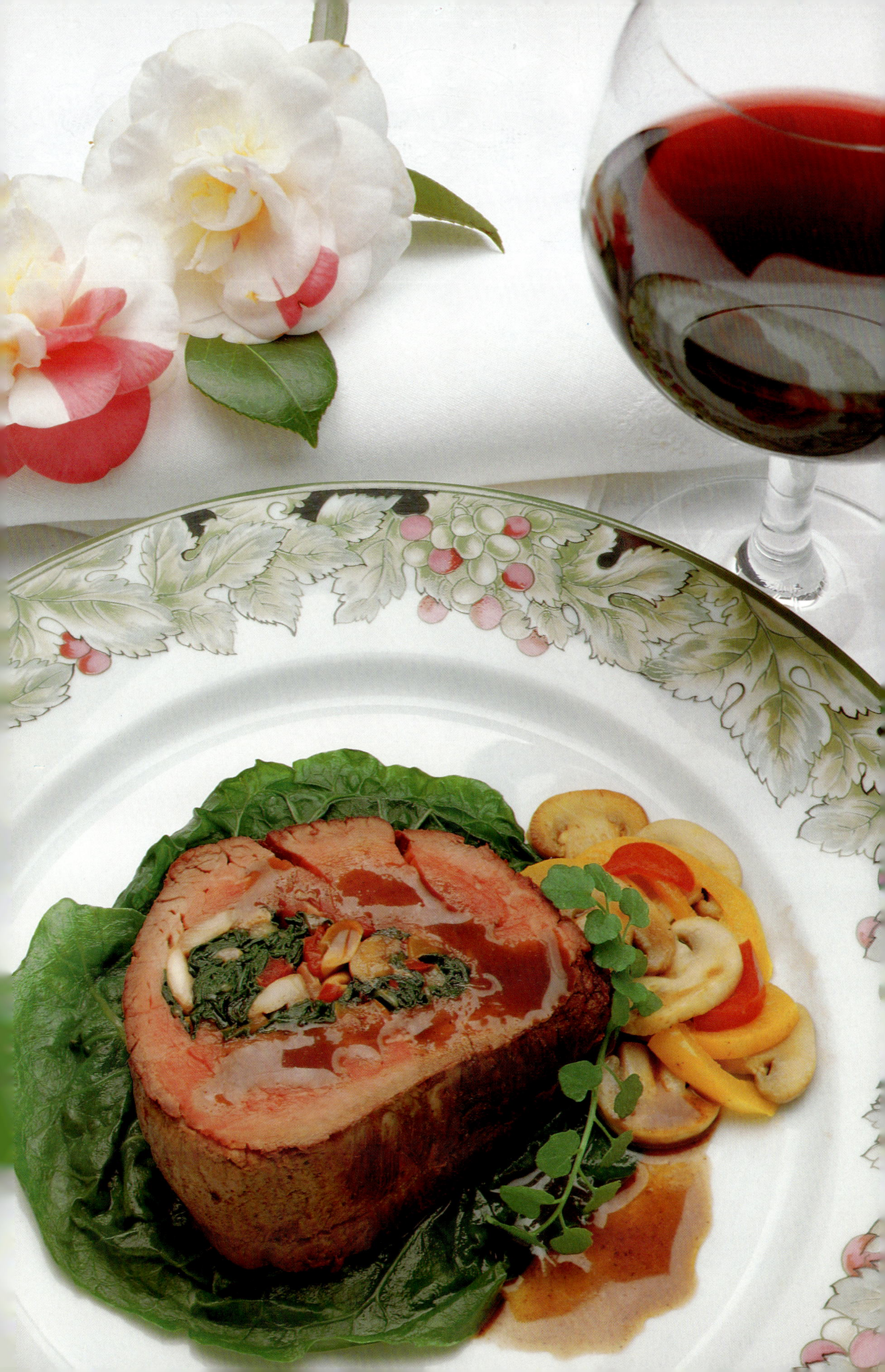

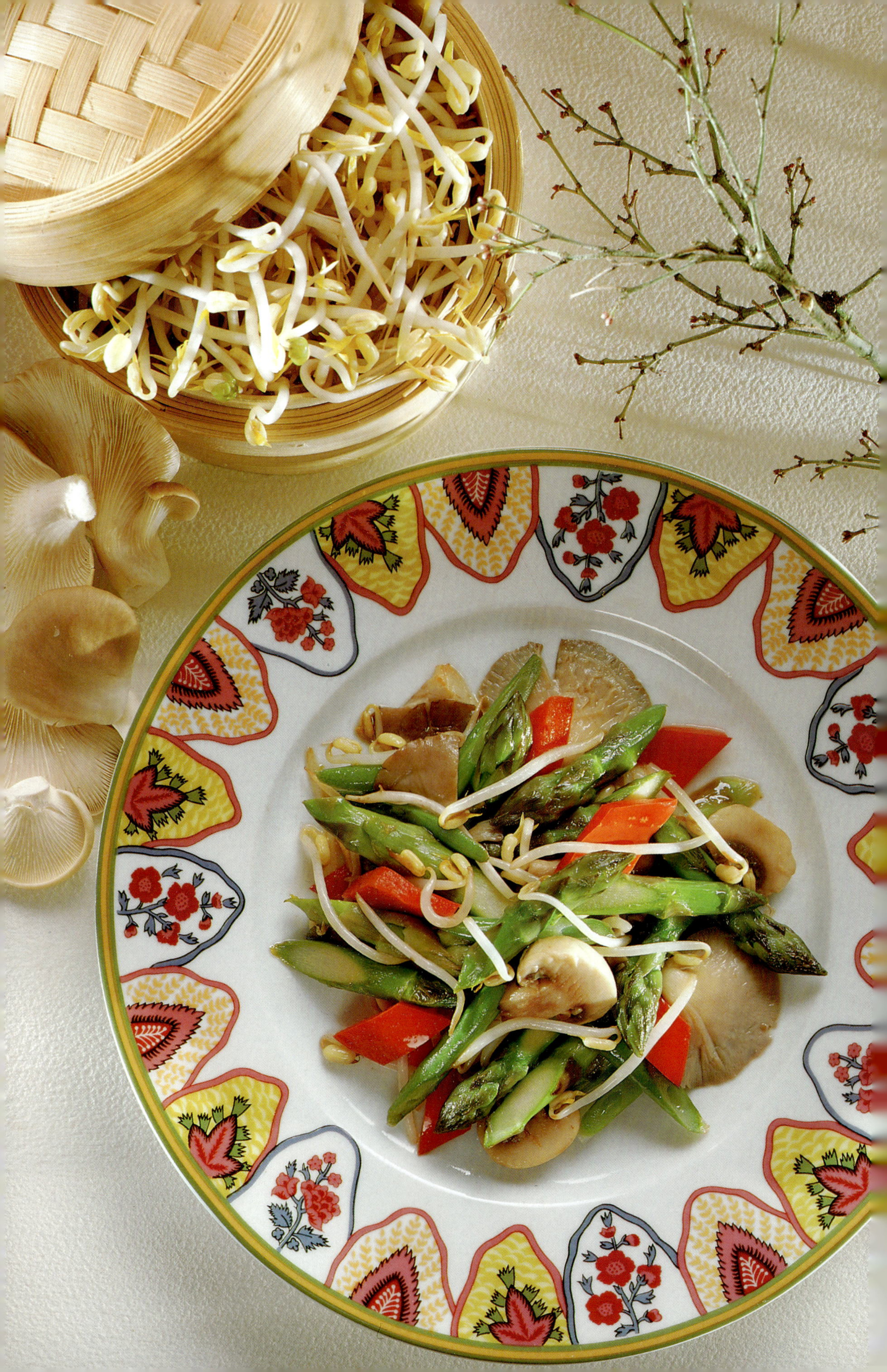

Stir-fried lamb with couscous

This exotic dish of North African flavours can be adapted to your family's taste by using spices and vegetables of your choice. Couscous, a coarse semolina that takes less time to prepare than rice, is available in most supermarkets.

SERVES ABOUT 4

1½ cups couscous

300 g (11 oz) deboned lean lamb from the leg

¼ tsp cummin

¼ tsp hot chilli paste

2 tomatoes

2 zucchini

1 capsicum

½ tbsp olive oil

Cook couscous according to packet instructions. It takes a few minutes. Keep couscous warm.

Trim lamb of all fat and cut into very thin bite-size strips. Mix lamb in a bowl with cummin and chilli paste.

Wash and dice tomatoes and zucchini.

Halve capsicum and remove seeds. Dice capsicum.

Heat oil in wok. Add lamb strips and stir-fry until meat has browned. Transfer meat to a plate. Add tomato, zucchini and capsicum to wok and cook on high heat for about 5 mins. Then return lamb to wok, stir well and serve on a bed of couscous.

Stir-fried beef with asparagus

When preparing a stir-fry dish such as this one you will get a better result and save time by selecting vegetables of similar size and by cutting the meat into regular pieces.

SERVES ABOUT 4

300 g (11 oz) rump steak

1 tbsp salt-reduced soy sauce

1 tbsp dry sherry

1 tsp cornflour

about 16 medium asparagus spears

about 100 g (3½ oz) bean sprouts

1 tbsp peanut oil

½ clove garlic, crushed

1 thin slice ginger

¼ cup water

1 tsp hot chilli paste (optional)

Trim beef of all fat and cut into bite-size strips. In a bowl mix beef with soy sauce, sherry and cornflour.

Peel asparagus starting from just below the tip and descending to the base. Then snap off the hard part at the base of the stalk. Steam or microwave asparagus for 2 mins then drain.

Wash bean sprouts and trim the roots.

Heat two-thirds of the oil in a wok. Add garlic, the whole slice of ginger and the beef and stir-fry until meat has browned. Transfer meat to a plate, discarding ginger.

Pour remaining oil into wok and stir-fry asparagus for about 15 secs. Add bean sprouts and stir-fry for a further 30 secs before pouring water down the inside of the wok. Stir well, cover and cook until asparagus is tender but still crunchy. Then add beef, stir well to reheat and serve.

Serve chilli paste separately.

SERVING SUGGESTION: Serve with Asian noodles or brown rice.

◁

Subtle flavours, wonderful texture – asparagus and mushrooms, sliced and stir-fried in minutes (page 32)

Pork bami in Rita's style

Our family and friends are a precious source of cooking ideas and recipes. Rita is a Dutch friend who lived in Indonesia and introduced Angie to bami and other Asian delights. Basically, bami is an Asian noodle dish with vegetables and whatever meat or seafood you fancy. It is one of our family treats and is best cooked in a wok. Once you have mastered the cutting technique, you'll zip through the preparation.

SERVES ABOUT 4

about 150 g (5 oz) Asian noodles

½ red capsicum

1 stick celery

1 medium carrot

½ brown onion

¼ cabbage

1 clove garlic

1 rasher bacon, trimmed of fat

1 tbsp peanut or polyunsaturated oil

200 g (7 oz) lean minced pork

100 g (3½ oz) shrimps

1 tsp grated ginger

1 tsp hot chilli paste

1 tbsp salt-reduced soy sauce

freshly ground black pepper

Cook noodles for 3 mins in boiling water then strain and refresh them under cold tap. Put aside.

Remove capsicum seeds. Wash and dice capsicum.

Dice celery, carrot and onion.

Wash and finely shred cabbage.

Chop garlic and bacon.

Heat wok for a few seconds then heat half the oil in the wok on high heat. Fry onion and bacon until onion just begins to brown around the edges. Using an egg lifter so as to leave as much oil in the wok as possible, transfer onion and bacon to a bowl.

Add garlic to wok, stir quickly then immediately add minced meat and shrimps. Loosen meat and stir-fry until brown. Transfer meat and shrimps to bowl with onion and bacon.

Add remaining oil to wok. Add ginger, capsicum, celery and carrot and stir-fry for about 30 secs. Then add cabbage and stir-fry until cabbage softens a little. Lastly, add noodles, meat, shrimps, onion and bacon, and season with chilli paste, soy sauce and a little pepper. Stir gently until reheated.

Serve immediately.

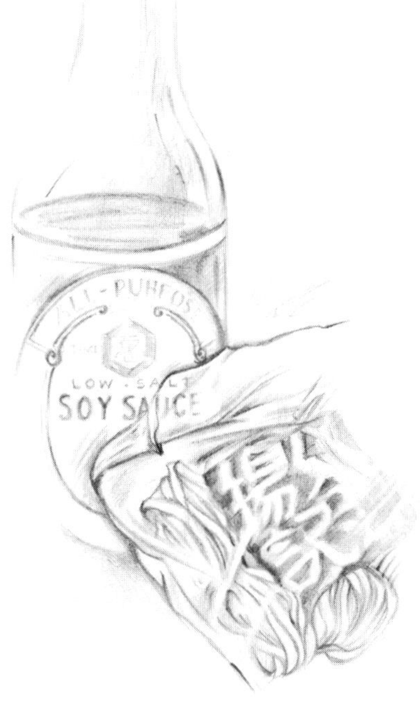

Spicy roast pork sirloin

Pork sirloin is an even cut that is very easy to carve into regular slices. Although the pork needs to be well cooked, it must not be dry. I have obtained the best results by calculating the cooking time to allow about 20 mins of roasting at 180°C/350°F for every 500 g (about 1 lb) of meat and then, after removal from the oven, allowing the roast to rest, covered with foil, for about 10 mins before carving it.

SERVES 4–6

1 tsp honey

¼ tsp hot chilli paste

½ tsp fennel seeds

½ tsp ground cummin

½ tsp paprika

1 tsp low-fat natural yoghurt

1 kg (about 2 lb) pork sirloin, trimmed of fat

1 small carrot, diced

½ onion, diced

½ cup white wine

½ cup water

freshly ground black pepper

Preheat oven to 220°C/450°F.

In a small bowl thoroughly mix honey, chilli paste, fennel seeds, ground cummin, paprika and yoghurt.

If you wish, tie the meat firmly with kitchen string. This helps the roast cook more regularly and retain its moisture. Rub or brush the roast all over with the spicy paste.

Place sirloin on an oven rack resting in an oven tray and add diced carrot and onion to tray. Place tray in preheated oven, reduce oven temperature to 180°C/350°F and roast for 30 mins.

Turn roast over and cook for a further 10 mins. Remove roast from oven, cover with foil or a lid and allow to rest for about 10 mins.

Drain fat from oven tray. Add wine to tray containing the carrot and onion and bring to boil for a few seconds. Add water, boil and reduce liquid by half. Season with a little pepper and strain into a small saucepan or sauce boat, discarding the carrot and onion.

Carve meat and serve with the sauce.

SERVING SUGGESTION: Serve with steamed bok choy and Asian noodles seasoned with a little salt-reduced soy sauce.

Roast beef with silver beet and mushrooms

Beef fillet is lean and very tender but, unfortunately, it is one of the most expensive cuts of meat, so perhaps this dish is a good one to choose for a special occasion. Select a regular piece of meat and ask your butcher to trim it of all fat, nerves and skin. This lovely dish is in the photograph opposite page 116.

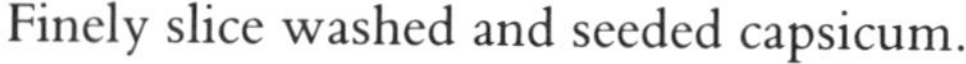

SERVES 4

½ red or yellow capsicum

400 g (14 oz) mushrooms

a little olive oil

1 bunch silver beet

½ cup water

freshly ground black pepper

1 clove garlic, chopped

2 tbsp chopped parsley

3 tbsp madeira or port

600 g (1¼ lb) beef fillet, in one piece

½ onion, diced

1 small carrot, diced

1 tsp cornflour mixed with 1 tbsp water

Finely slice washed and seeded capsicum.

Wash mushrooms briefly then slice them.

Brush a large saucepan with a little oil and on high heat cook capsicum for 1 min, stirring with a wooden spoon. Add mushroom and cook for 3 to 4 mins.

Discard any damaged silver beet leaves then separate the green leaves from the stalks, keeping the stalks for another vegetable dish. Wash silver beet several times in cold water. Add silver beet and ½ cup water to capsicum and mushroom, cover pan and cook for a few minutes until silver beet has softened. Transfer vegetables to a bowl, reserving the liquid for the sauce. Season vegetables with pepper, garlic, parsley and 1 tbsp of the madeira.

Using a sharp knife and starting from the smaller end of the fillet, make a small incision in the meat. Don't slit right through to the other end. Just make a long pocket. Fill this pocket with about 5 tbsp of the mushroom and silver beet preparation (there will be some left over). Tie fillet with a few rounds of kitchen string and season meat with pepper. Preheat oven to 180°C/350°F.

Brush a small, heavy roasting tray with a little olive oil and on high heat brown beef on all sides. Add diced onion and carrot and place in preheated oven. Bake for 15 to 20 mins, depending on how you prefer your beef. Place cooked beef on a warm serving platter, cover with foil or a lid and leave to rest.

Place roasting tray on medium heat and stir-fry onion and carrot for 1 min. Add remaining madeira, bring to boil and add mushroom and silver beet juice. Return to boil, cook for 3 mins then strain sauce into a smaller saucepan, discarding onion and carrot.

Reheat remaining capsicum, mushroom and silver beet.

Bring strained sauce to boil and stir in cornflour mixed with 1 tbsp water. When the sauce has thickened a little, season it well with pepper.

Carve roast into four slices and serve with the vegetables and sauce.

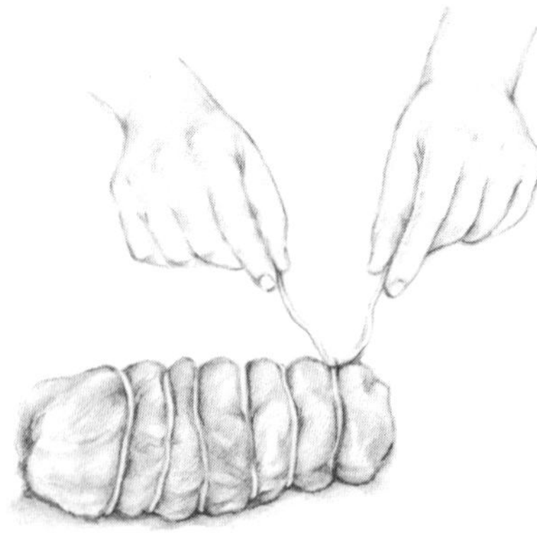

Roast boned leg of lamb

A roast boned leg of lamb takes less time to cook and is much easier to slice than a roast on the bone. Ask your butcher to trim the leg of as much fat as possible and to roll the roast into a regular shape and tie it with string. My local butcher doesn't mind doing this but prefers the order to be placed in advance.

SERVES 6–8

2 cloves garlic

**1 medium boned rolled
leg of lamb**

1 tbsp olive oil

**1 tsp finely chopped lemon
thyme or rosemary**

freshly ground black pepper

1 medium carrot

1 small brown onion

½ cup dry white wine

½ cup water

Preheat oven to 220°C/450°F.

Peel garlic and cut each clove into four. Using the tip of the blade of a small knife, make eight small cuts in the lamb, deep enough to insert a piece of garlic. The garlic must not protrude from the meat.

In a bowl mix olive oil, lemon thyme and a little pepper then brush meat all over with this mixture. Place lamb on a rack and set the rack in a roasting tray.

Peel and dice carrot and onion and mix them in the bowl used previously. There should be some oil mixture remaining to coat the vegetables lightly. Place vegetables in roasting tray with the meat and bake in oven. After 10 mins turn meat over and reduce temperature to about 150°C/300°F. Roast for a further 30 mins before adding wine and water to roasting tray and turning meat over again. Roast for a further 10 to 20 mins, depending on the size of your roast and on how you like your meat done.

An easy method of checking whether the meat is cooked is to use a meat thermometer, which registers the temperature at the centre of the meat. The markings on the thermometer indicate what temperature is appropriate for each type of roast meat. I like my roast to be pink in the centre and so cook it until the thermometer reads about 70°C/160°F (although my thermometer suggests a slightly higher temperature is best).

Remove roast from oven and place meat on a serving dish. Cover with foil and leave to rest for about 10 mins.

Strain gravy from roasting tray into a small saucepan, discarding vegetables. Bring gravy to a simmer and season to taste with a little pepper. Remove fat from the top using a spoon or gravy skimmer and if the meat has released any juices, add them to your gravy.

Remove string from meat. Slice roast and serve with hot gravy.

SERVING SUGGESTION: Serve with roast vegetables, cooked in a separate dish, and green vegetables.

Roast veal and mushroom sauce

This roast is easy to prepare, cook, carve and serve, and the mushroom sauce has a lovely balance of flavours. A rolled veal roast may not always be readily available, so ask your butcher in advance to prepare one for you, indicating the weight you require, and order a piece from the neck or shoulder, which is more suitable for roasting than other cuts. To roast veal, I use a thick ovenproof casserole dish with a lid.

SERVES 4–6

½ tbsp olive oil

1 kg (about 2 lb) rolled roast veal

2 sprigs lemon thyme, chopped

1 small carrot, diced

½ onion, diced

½ cup dry white wine

2 peeled tomatoes (from a can), chopped

1 clove garlic, left whole

250 g (9 oz) mushrooms, sliced

freshly ground black pepper

2 tbsp chopped parsley

Preheat oven to 180°C/350°F.

Brush stove-top casserole dish with oil and heat it on top of stove. Brown veal on all sides. Add chopped thyme, diced carrot and onion. Place dish, uncovered, in oven and roast for 30 mins, turning the veal once. Add wine, tomato and garlic, cover and bake for a further 20 mins.

Remove dish from oven and place roast veal on a serving dish. Cover with foil or a lid and allow roast to rest for 10 mins before serving.

Meanwhile, bring sauce in casserole to boil and strain it into a smaller saucepan, discarding carrot and onion. Add mushroom to casserole dish and cook on medium heat for 2 mins, stirring continuously. Add sauce to dish and stir for 1 min before seasoning with pepper and stirring in parsley.

Remove string from roast, carve meat and serve with the sauce.

SERVING SUGGESTION: Serve with boiled potatoes and steamed beans.

Fast Finales

Of all the recipes that I have demonstrated on television or broadcast on radio over the last ten years, it is the desserts – and particularly the fast ones – that have always been the most popular. We all seem to have a sweet tooth, which is hardly surprising when you think that the sweet milk of our mothers was for many of us our very first food. People often ask me if desserts are bad for us. They need not be as long as we limit our consumption of fat and sugar, for these can have a negative effect on our health.

Many traditional desserts are rich. There is no need to worry about having an occasional slice of chocolate cake or a vanilla slice. However, on a daily basis, if we wish to include desserts in our diet, we need to choose those that are low in added fat and sugar. There are several concerns about eating food that is high in added sugar. One problem, which must not be under-estimated, is that sugar promotes tooth decay. People with bad teeth have problems chewing food properly. Food lovers value their teeth.

Sugar is also high in kilojoules (calories), so reduced consumption helps to keep the weight down and, therefore, may reduce the risk of diseases such as cancer, heart disease and diabetes.

In this chapter many desserts are prepared without added fat and sugar and are, at the same time, a good source of nutrients, such as fibre, vitamins and minerals, including calcium. Many of the fastest recipes use fresh fruits. Treat yourself, your family and your friends to seasonal fruits, which are usually cheaper and sweeter than fruits out of season, and remember to keep a good variety in your fruit bowl – a piece of fruit in between meals is an excellent snack. Our children enjoy fruit salad for dessert, especially when we include something special like cherries, apricots, nectarines, mangoes and mandarins as a change from the more common apples, bananas and oranges.

Cooked fruits are also very satisfying. Baked apples, pears and nashis, one of the newer fruits in our markets, are really delicious. Don't forget about poached fruits; peaches, apples, pears, apricots and red fruits are all beautiful when poached. You might like to try our recipe for poached figs and red plums with spices. There are also special dishes, such as pancakes, crumbles and strudels, which can be prepared using a minimal amount of fat and are crammed with good things.

Low-fat dairy products are a good source of much-needed calcium, and in the preparation of your everyday desserts you should use low-fat milk rather than full-cream milk. Our family enjoys natural low-fat yoghurt and fresh low-fat cheese, which we whip into a smooth, creamy consistency with a little low-fat milk and 1 tsp of sugar. The fresh, low-fat cheese referred to and used frequently in this book is the Australian version of the German quark or the French fromage blanc and comes with a milk-fat content of less than 8 per cent and sometimes as low as 0.2 per cent. Ask at your supermarket or local deli for it.

Restrict rich icecreams and cream to special occasions and use them in moderate quantities. Remember that for a special occasion your family and guests will appreciate a rich dessert only after a light meal. After a rich meal most people prefer a light dessert.

Blueberry and raspberry sauce

The availability of blueberries has increased markedly in the last few years. As with grapes, such as Pinot Noir, much of their flavour and colour comes from the skin rather than from the pulp. You can substitute blueberries and raspberries with other berries in this quick and easy preparation ideally served with pudding, fruit compote or cake, or with sliced fruit such as peaches for a quick but delicious dessert.

SERVES ABOUT 6

½ **cup blueberries**

½ **cup raspberries**

juice of 1 orange

juice of ½ lemon

1 tbsp castor sugar

Blend washed blueberries and unwashed raspberries with orange and lemon juice and castor sugar. Strain through a sieve to discard berry seeds. Refrigerate until a little while before using.

Apricot and almond sauce

Apricot is a favourite fruit because it has a beautiful balance of sweetness and acidity. This sauce is excellent as an accompaniment to fruit loaves, cakes and baked fruit. You need to prepare it in advance as the dried apricots need to be boiled and cooled.

SERVES ABOUT 4

12 dried apricots

1 tsp finely grated orange or mandarin rind

½ cup water

6 raw almonds

juice of ½ lemon

2 drops vanilla essence

1 tbsp Kirsch or Drambuie or Cointreau (optional)

Place apricots and orange rind in ½ cup water, bring to boil, cover and simmer for about 3 mins. Allow to cool.

Chop almonds finely.

Blend apricots and liquid to a smooth purée. Stir in lemon juice, vanilla essence, chopped almonds and liqueur. The sauce should be runny, so add a little fruit juice such as orange or apple, if necessary, to make it more runny.

Delicious creamy topping

This creamy topping, made of fresh low-fat soft cheese, can be whipped up in seconds. It is a lovely alternative to cream or icecream to go with desserts, such as fruit salads, pancakes, strudels, etc. Manufacturers have varying names for this type of fresh low-fat soft cheese but it is similar to the German quark or the French fromage blanc. Ask your local delicatessen for it. The topping is especially lovely with fruit crumble, as in our photograph opposite page 132.

SERVES ABOUT 4–6

5 tbsp quark (fresh low-fat soft cheese with a milk-fat content of less than 8 per cent)

3 tbsp low-fat milk

1 tsp castor sugar or honey

a pinch of ground cinnamon or 2 drops vanilla essence or 1 tsp grated lemon, orange or mandarin rind

Blend or whisk all ingredients to a creamy consistency and refrigerate if not using immediately.

Orange and polenta custard

This runny custard can be served with fresh fruit, cake or pudding. If you prefer it thicker, increase the quantity of polenta. Polenta is a corn meal, much used in Italian cooking. It has a yellow colour and its thickening qualities make it a good alternative to an egg custard.

SERVES 6

1½ tbsp polenta

1½ cups low-fat milk

1 tbsp finely grated orange rind

1 tbsp sugar or honey

½ tsp vanilla essence

In a small bowl combine polenta with 2 tbsp of the milk until a paste is formed. This takes about 20 secs.

Slightly heat remaining milk and orange rind, then add polenta, sugar and vanilla and slowly bring to boil. Boil for 1 min, stirring continuously. The custard thickens a little. The first time you prepare polenta you may be surprised at the tiny lumps, but this is the way it should be and there is no need to strain it.

Serve hot or transfer to a bowl to cool.

Apple muffins

The secret of a good muffin is speed – the faster you prepare muffins the better they taste. Our children particularly like apple muffins.

MAKES ABOUT 12 MUFFINS

a little melted margarine

1 large apple, Granny Smith or Golden Delicious

3 tbsp sultanas

a pinch of cinnamon

2 tbsp honey

1½ tbsp polyunsaturated oil

¾ cup low-fat milk

1 cup wholemeal self-raising flour

½ cup white self-raising flour

Brush muffin tray with melted margarine.

Preheat oven to 200°C/400°F.

Peel, core and dice apple. Place apple in a bowl with sultanas, cinnamon, honey, oil and milk. Gently mix to dilute honey.

Place the two types of flour in a large bowl. Pour the apple and liquid preparation onto the flour and, using a wooden spoon, stir until just combined. It is important not to overmix. Spoon this preparation immediately into your muffin tins and bake in preheated oven for 15 to 20 mins. When cooked, turn muffins out onto a wire rack.

Rhubarb sorbet

Though its peak season is in the warmest months of the year, rhubarb is available all year round. This sorbet is delicious on its own or with stewed berries. If your family enjoys icecream and sorbets like mine does, you will find an icecream maker a great timesaver.

SERVES 8

5 cups diced, peeled rhubarb

1½ cups water

4 tbsp sugar

1 tsp grated lemon rind

1 tsp grated orange rind

juice of ½ lemon

a pinch of cinnamon

4 drops vanilla essence

Place rhubarb in a saucepan with water, sugar and lemon and orange rind. Bring to a gentle boil, cover and simmer until rhubarb is just soft. It takes about 5 to 10 mins. Allow to cool.

Add lemon juice, cinnamon and vanilla essence, and blend rhubarb and liquid to a very fine purée. Place purée in icecream maker and make your sorbet. Store in the freezer in a covered bowl or in an icecream container with lid.

If you don't have an icecream maker, place preparation in a stainless-steel bowl in freezer. When purée starts to set, whisk for 10 to 15 secs and return bowl to freezer. Repeat this procedure until the purée is too hard to whisk. The whisking lightens the sorbet.

Granny Smith sorbet

I first made this sorbet to accompany the nutty cherry and apple strudel described in this chapter. It is lovely both by itself and as an accompaniment to desserts that go well with icecream. You will get better results if you use an icecream maker.

SERVES 8

4 Granny Smith apples

1½ cups water

¼ tsp cinnamon

3 drops vanilla essence

4 tbsp sugar

grated rind of ½ lemon

juice of ½ lemon

Peel, quarter and core apples and place them in a saucepan with water, cinnamon, vanilla essence, sugar, grated lemon rind and lemon juice. Bring to boil, cover and cook until apples are soft. Blend apples and liquid to a very fine purée and allow to cool.

Place cold apple purée in icecream maker and make your sorbet. Store in the freezer in a covered bowl or in an icecream container with lid.

If you don't have an icecream maker, place preparation in a stainless-steel bowl in freezer. When the purée starts to set, whisk it for 10 to 15 secs and return bowl to freezer. Repeat this procedure until the purée is too hard to whisk. The whisking lightens the sorbet.

William pear sorbet

William pears are best in the autumn months when their sweet perfume is most charming.

SERVES 8

5 William pears
1½ cups water
juice of 1 lemon
4 tbsp sugar
grated rind of ½ lemon
3 drops vanilla essence

Peel, quarter and core pears. Place in a saucepan with water, half of the lemon juice, sugar and lemon rind. Bring to a gentle boil, cover and simmer for about 10 mins or until pears are just soft. Allow to cool. Add remaining lemon juice and vanilla essence, and blend pears and liquid to a very fine purée.

Place purée in icecream maker and make your sorbet. Store in the freezer in a covered bowl or in an icecream container with lid.

If you don't have an icecream maker, place preparation in a stainless-steel bowl in freezer. When purée starts to set, whisk it for 10 to 15 secs and return to freezer. Repeat this procedure until the purée is too hard to whisk. The whisking lightens the sorbet.

Quick peach fantasy

This smooth family dessert is a tribute to the genuine effort being made by the food industry to provide tasty foods that are low in fat and sugar. It can be whipped up in an instant, so it is perfect for midweek meals.

SERVES ABOUT 4

a 425 g (15 oz) can peach slices in natural juice
250 g (9 oz) quark (cheese)

Drain peach slices and blend juice with the soft cheese until well mixed and very smooth. Place this cream in a bowl, stir in peach slices and refrigerate until required.

Barbecued fruit kebabs

Children love preparing kebabs and this is a dish to which they can safely contribute. If using bamboo or wooden sticks, first soak them in water for 30 mins to prevent them from burning on the barbecue. The kebabs can also be cooked under the grill, in the oven or in a pan. They are easier to cook when all the fruit is cut about the same size. These kebabs are also delicious eaten raw if the kids can't wait.

MAKES ABOUT 12 KEBABS

3 kiwi fruits
½ pineapple
4 bananas

Peel and quarter kiwi fruits. Peel, quarter and core pineapple and cut into regular pieces. Peel bananas and cut into regular pieces.

Alternately thread fruit onto kebabs, leaving no gaps in between.

Cook on a clean, hot barbecue for about 6 mins, remembering to turn kebabs over halfway through cooking.

Peaches and red fruit salad

This luscious, tangy dessert is very popular as a finish to a special meal and is quick and easy to prepare. It is light and leaves the most beautiful aftertaste. Quel souvenir! The dish is shown in the photograph opposite page 20.

SERVES 6–8

250 g (9 oz) raspberries

1 tbsp castor sugar

juice of 2 oranges

juice of ½ lemon

2 cups berries (blueberries, blackberries, strawberries or other available berries)

4 ripe peaches or a 400 g (14 oz) can peach halves, drained

2 tbsp Drambuie (optional)

12 raw almonds, cut into small pieces

Blend raspberries, sugar and citrus juices to a purée. Pass blended fruit through a fine strainer into an attractive bowl.

Wash strawberries and blueberries, if using, leaving other berries unwashed.

Gently stir berries into raspberry sauce.

Wash peaches gently. Halve peaches and cut them into segments about 1 cm (⅓ in) thick. Add peaches to bowl as you slice them. Gently stir to coat peach slices with red sauce.

Refrigerate fruit salad if not using within 30 mins, but it is best served at room temperature.

Stir in Drambuie and almond pieces just before serving.

Tropical fruit salad

This is a fruit salad for all occasions but at home we enjoy it especially after spicy food or as a way of showing off the culinary delights of Australia to overseas visitors.

SERVES 6

2 slices pineapple, 1 cm (⅓ in) thick

juice of 2 oranges

2 passionfruits

1 tbsp sugar

2 bananas

¼ small pawpaw

1 small custard apple

6 rambutans or lychees

Trim and core pineapple and blend to a liquid with orange juice. Place in a bowl and add passionfruit pulp, sugar, sliced bananas, and peeled and sliced pawpaw.

Open custard apple and gently scoop out the white flesh, avoiding the mushy pulp just under the skin. Discard seeds and add custard apple to bowl.

Peel and stone rambutans and add to bowl.

Refrigerate fruit salad. Remove from refrigerator at least 20 mins before serving to allow the fruits to return to room temperature.

Rhubarb and blackberry crumble

A fruit crumble is a treat and full of goodness. The main fruit here is rhubarb but you can also use apricots, pears and berries. Rhubarb is available throughout the year but is at its peak in summer. The crumble is cooked in a gratin or oven dish big enough to serve six people, and it is shown in the photograph opposite page 132.

SERVES 6

3 cups diced, peeled rhubarb

1 tbsp grated orange rind

1 apple

1 tbsp water

1 tbsp castor sugar

6 tbsp rolled oats

1 tbsp plain wholemeal flour

1 tbsp desiccated coconut

1 tbsp chopped raw almonds

1 tbsp polyunsaturated margarine or butter

1 tbsp honey

250 g (9 oz) blackberries (or other berries)

Place rhubarb and rind in a saucepan with peeled, quartered and diced apple and the water. Cook on medium heat until apple and rhubarb are just soft. Stir in castor sugar.

Thoroughly combine rolled oats, flour, coconut, almonds, margarine and honey. This is best done by hand.

Preheat oven to 210°C/430°F.

Spoon apple and rhubarb into oven dish and top with blackberries. Spread crumble mixture over fruit and pat down a little. Place dish in oven and cook for 10 to 15 mins or until the top is golden brown.

Serve hot or cold.

Winter fruit compote in wine

Although served cold, this dessert is warm in flavour with sweet spices and wine, and is ideal for a Sunday lunch. I love the aroma that this dish creates in the kitchen when it is cooking. Use a saucepan just large enough to hold the fruit. If your pantry cupboard is well stocked, all you need are fresh pears and an orange, so this dish is fantastic for spontaneous entertaining.

SERVES 4

4 small pears

1 orange

12 moist prunes

a 2.5 cm (1 in) stick cinnamon

2 coriander seeds

1 clove

¼ bay leaf (optional)

⅓ vanilla pod

4 tbsp castor sugar

1½ cups good red wine

Peel pears, and wash and cut orange into ½ cm (¼ in) slices.

Gently place pears stalk end up in saucepan. Place prunes in between pears and add cinnamon, coriander seeds, clove, bay leaf, vanilla and castor sugar. Top with orange slices and add wine. If necessary add water so that there is just enough liquid to cover the fruit.

Bring to boil, lower to a simmer, and poach pears for 25 to 30 mins until soft. Leave fruit to cool in liquid.

Remove spices and serve fruit and liquid from an attractive serving dish.

Poached figs and red plums with spices

This is an autumn treat, a luscious dessert to cap off a lovely dinner party. You might like to serve it with a berry sauce such as the blueberry and raspberry sauce in this chapter. Other fruits such as peaches, apricots, nashis, apples and pears can be used. I prefer this dessert cold and it makes a delicious breakfast, too.

SERVES 4

4 cups water

2 tbsp castor sugar

¼ vanilla pod

a 2.5 cm (1 in) stick cinnamon

grated rind of 1 orange and ½ lemon

1 clove

8 red plums

4 figs, ripe but not too soft

Pour water into a large saucepan and add sugar, vanilla, cinnamon, orange and lemon rind, and clove. Bring to boil and simmer for 10 mins to allow the spices to flavour the water.

Wash and halve plums and remove stones. Add plums to infusion and poach them in the simmering liquid for 5 mins.

Gently wash figs, add to saucepan and simmer together with plums for a further 10 mins.

Leave fruits to cool in liquid then serve at room temperature.

Baked nashis with exotic fruits

Nashis are an autumn and winter fruit, very popular with Asian people. They are juicy, like pears, but have more of a crunchy apple texture, and are beautiful when baked. Select them firm, but not too firm. The colour should be green turning to yellow. Preparation time is minimal, but allow 45 mins to 1 hr to cook.

SERVES 4

4 nashis

2 bananas

4 dried apricots

4 almonds

1 tbsp diced dried mango

½ cup apple juice (or other juice or water)

1 tbsp sugar

2 passionfruits

Preheat oven to 180°C/350°F.

Wash and core nashis. Dice bananas and apricots and chop almonds coarsely. Mix in a bowl with diced mango.

Place nashis in an oven dish just large enough to hold them. Fill nashis with fruit mixture, spooning any remaining fruit into the base of the dish. Pour apple juice over nashis and sprinkle them with sugar.

Bake in oven for 45 mins to 1 hr reducing temperature if the top of the fruit colours too much. Test whether the fruit is cooked by piercing one of the nashis with the blade of a small knife. It should feel soft.

Transfer nashis onto serving plate. Stir passionfruit pulp into the fruit remaining in dish and spoon this over nashis.

Mandarin pancakes

Pancakes would have to rate on the top-ten dessert list of most children. Filled with fresh or canned fruit, with cooked apple, pear or rhubarb, pancakes do not require cream or icecream when served as a family dessert. Use a small, flat, smooth frying pan with an unscratched surface. Make the batter before dinner, as it needs to stand for at least 30 mins before cooking. For a special occasion, serve the pancakes as in our photograph opposite page 5.

MAKES ABOUT 6 PANCAKES

½ cup plain white flour

½ cup plain wholemeal flour

1 egg

1½ cups low-fat milk

a small pinch of salt

1 tsp grated mandarin rind

6 mandarins

1 tbsp castor sugar

1 tsp peanut oil

1 tsp polyunsaturated margarine or butter

a little icing sugar from a shaker (optional)

Place both types of flour in a bowl and make a hollow in the centre. Into the hollow pour egg and half of the milk. Add the salt and grated mandarin rind. Using a whisk, first mix egg and milk together then gradually incorporate flour, slowly adding the rest of the milk to form a smooth mixture. Refrigerate for at least 30 mins before using.

Juice two mandarins and segment the other four. Bring juice and sugar to boil for 2 mins, then add mandarin segments.

Heat oil and margarine in frying pan and when margarine has melted, pour it into pancake batter and mix well. This makes the batter lighter and helps prevent sticking.

Return pan to heat and, using a ladle, thinly cover bottom of pan with batter. Twirl pan smoothly to form a thin, even pancake.

When the upper half of pancake starts to dry, turn pancake over using a wide spatula. After browning the second side, remove pancake and start cooking another immediately, without adding any more margarine or oil to pan.

Spoon about four mandarin segments with a little juice onto each pancake and roll the pancakes up neatly. Place on a serving dish, reheat in the oven, and dust with a little icing sugar just before serving.

▷

Delicious rhubarb and blackberry crumble – an old-fashioned pudding to make in no time at all (page 130) with a lovely creamy topping (page 125)

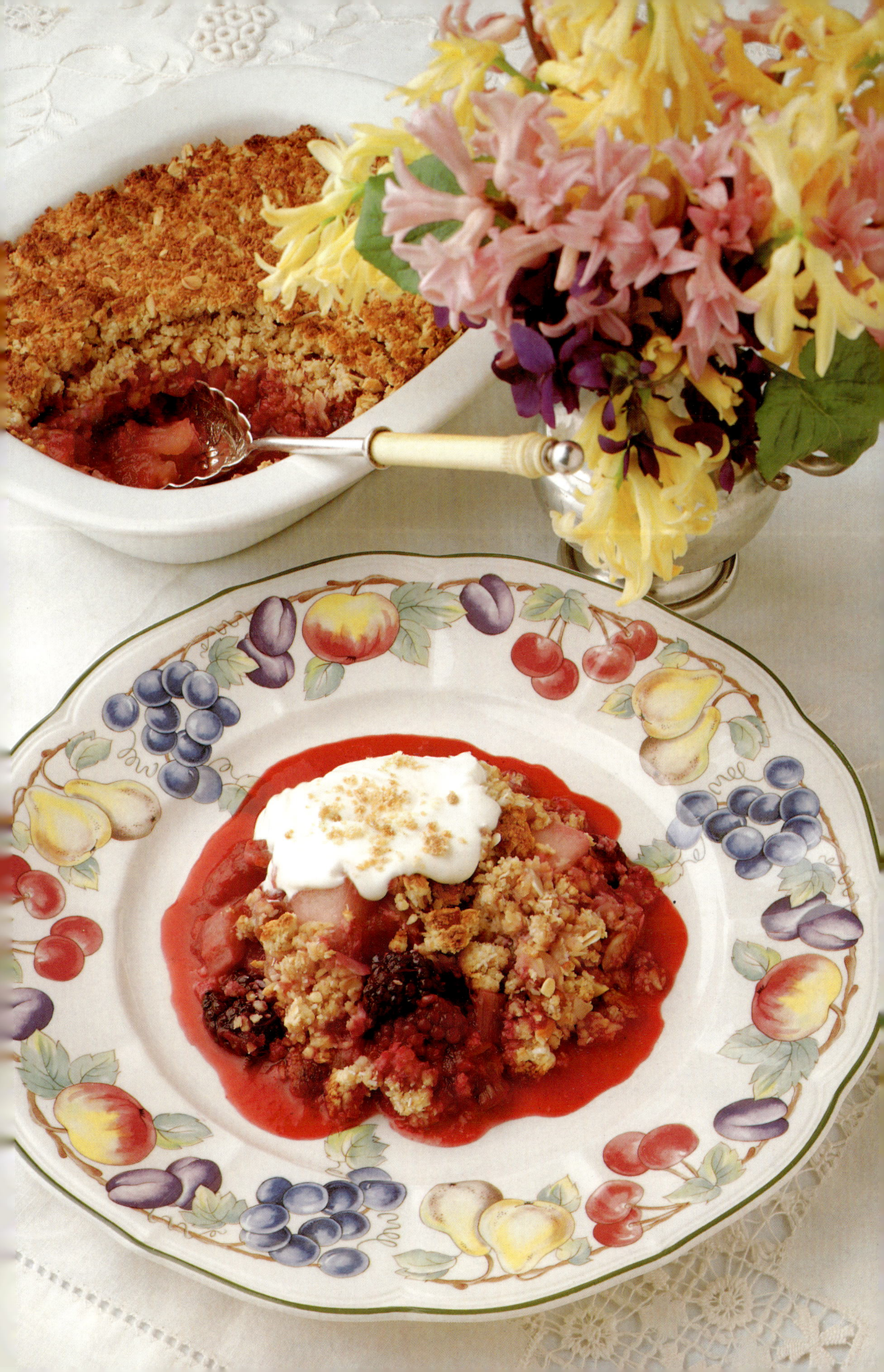

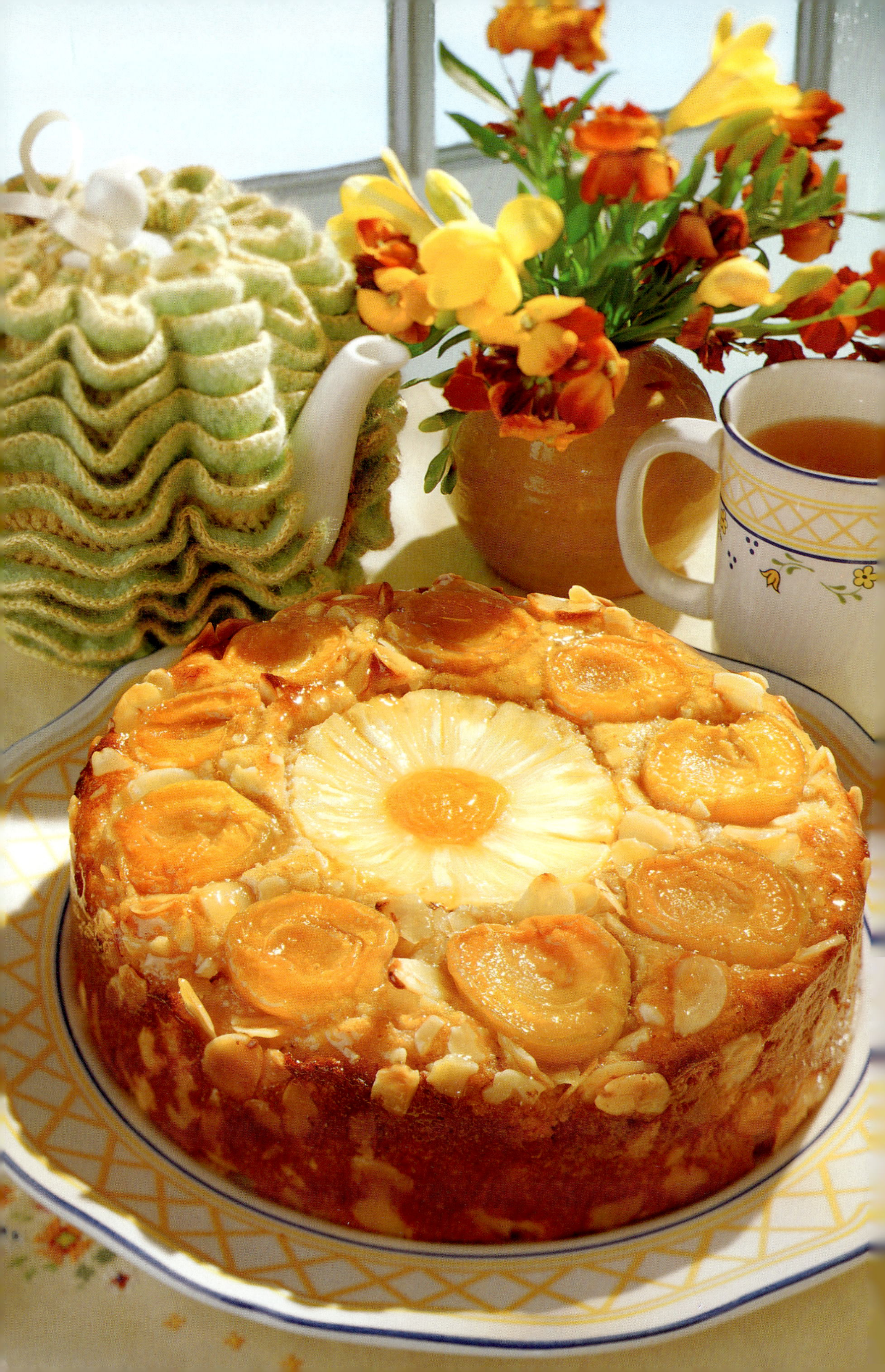

Pawpaw, mango and apricot loaf

This exotic, moist fruit cake is best cooked in a greased rectangular loaf tin. It contains no added sugar or fat but is rich, and a small slice is satisfying.

MAKES ABOUT 12 SLICES

200 g (7 oz) diced, dried pawpaw

200 g (7 oz) dried mango

20 dried apricots

5 dried pear halves

2 cups water

2 medium bananas

2 cups wholemeal self-raising flour

½ cup chopped raw almonds

¼ tsp cinnamon

Place dried pawpaw, mango, apricots and pears in a saucepan with the water. Bring to boil and simmer for about 5 mins. Strain off liquid and blend it with 10 of the apricots and the bananas to a fine purée.

Preheat oven to 180°C/350°F.

Transfer fruit purée to a mixing bowl and incorporate flour, almonds and cinnamon. Spoon a quarter of this cake mixture into greased loaf tin. Top with half of pawpaw and mango, then add another quarter of cake mixture. Top with remaining whole apricots and pears, then add another quarter of cake mixture. Top with remaining pawpaw and mango and finish with remaining cake mixture.

Tap tin to ensure that it is properly filled and flatten top of the mixture using a wet spoon.

Bake in oven for about 50 mins. Allow to cool a little before unmoulding onto a cake rack.

Serve with a berry sauce such as the blueberry and raspberry sauce in this chapter.

French filo apple tart

A French apple tart is often made with puff pastry, but for this one I use the much lighter filo pastry and the result is lovely.

SERVES ABOUT 6

5 Granny Smith apples

2 tbsp water

3 sheets of wholemeal filo pastry

a little peanut oil

1 tbsp low-fat cream

1 tbsp castor sugar

2 tbsp apricot jam or a little icing sugar from a shaker (optional)

◁

Sunshine-fresh fruits of apricot, banana and pineapple in a special-occasion gâteau (page 134)

Peel, quarter and core one apple and cook with 2 tbsp water in a covered pan until apple is soft. Mash apple and allow purée to cool. (If you spread it on a plate, it will cool more quickly.)

Peel, halve and core remaining four apples. Cut thinly into 2 mm (¹⁄₁₀ in) slices.

Line a baking sheet with 1 sheet of filo pastry. Brush it with a little oil and place another sheet of pastry on top. Again brush with oil and place a third sheet of pastry on top. Preheat oven to 220°C/450°F.

Stir cream into cold apple purée and spread this over pastry. Beginning at one corner, place apple slices on top of purée. The apple slices should overlap so as to leave no gaps and you'll probably have some apple left over. Sprinkle apple slices with castor sugar and cook in a hot oven for 15 mins. The pastry should be crisp and the edges of the apple slightly browned.

Before serving, brush with warm apricot jam or dust with icing sugar.

Apricot, banana and pineapple gâteau

This family gâteau has no added fat and very little added sugar. As the apricot season is very short, I use apricot halves canned in natural juice. If using fresh apricots, replace this juice with a fresh fruit juice such as apple or pear juice. To bake the gâteau you need a greased 20 cm (8 in) cake tin. It is illustrated opposite page 133.

SERVES 6–10

3 slices of pineapple, canned or fresh

1 medium ripe banana

a 425 g (15 oz) can apricot halves in natural juice, or 8 fresh apricots

1 tbsp honey

1 cup wholemeal self-raising flour

½ cup almond meal

2 egg whites

a pinch of salt

3 tbsp slivered almonds

1 tbsp smooth apricot jam or a little icing sugar

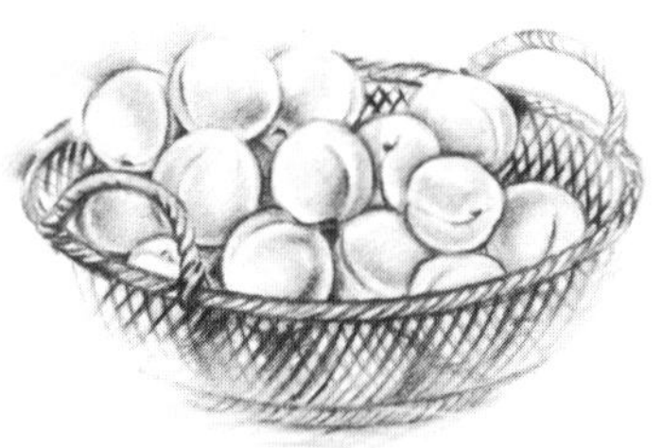

Preheat oven to 180°C/350°F.

Dice two slices of pineapple and place in a mixing bowl.

Blend banana, four apricot halves and 4 tbsp natural juice from the can (or 4 tbsp fresh fruit juice if using fresh apricots), to a smooth purée. Mix purée with diced pineapple then mix in honey, flour and almond meal.

Beat egg whites, with a pinch of salt added, to stiff peaks. Gently fold beaten egg white into cake preparation but don't overmix.

Sprinkle half of the slivered almonds into the bottom of the greased cake tin and pour cake preparation into tin. Smooth the top using the back of a soup spoon and sprinkle with remaining almonds. Place remaining pineapple slice in the centre, pushing it down slightly. Arrange remaining apricot halves around pineapple with the insides facing upwards, and again push them down slightly into the cake mixture.

Bake cake in preheated oven for 25 mins.

When cooked, remove cake from oven and leave to cool for a few minutes before carefully unmoulding onto a plate. Immediately place cake bottom down onto a cake rack.

Melt apricot jam in a small saucepan and brush over cake. Alternatively, dust cake with icing sugar.

Rhubarb and pear soufflé

This is our elder son's favourite soufflé. It is very light, and the blend of rhubarb and pear is truly magnificent. If you plan to serve this for a special occasion and it is your first attempt at making soufflé, you may like to practise on your family first. Making a soufflé is not so hard, and it is one of the most impressive of all desserts.

SERVES 4

a little polyunsaturated margarine or butter

a little castor sugar

1 pear (William pears are excellent)

1 cup diced, peeled rhubarb

1 tbsp water

a few drops lemon juice

1 tsp grated orange rind

2 tbsp castor sugar

4 egg whites

a pinch of salt

a little icing sugar (from a shaker)

Grease four individual soufflé moulds with a little margarine and dust with castor sugar.

Peel, quarter and core pear. Cut pear into small pieces and place in a saucepan with rhubarb. Add water, lemon juice and grated orange rind. Cover and cook until fruits are soft. Blend fruit to a fine purée. Add 1 tbsp castor sugar and stir on low heat for about 2 mins to evaporate a little moisture from fruit. Transfer purée to a mixing bowl.

Preheat oven to 180°C/350°F.

In a medium mixing bowl, beat egg whites with a pinch of salt added, and when the whites are almost firm, add remaining 1 tbsp castor sugar. Continue beating until whites are stiff.

Mix about one-third of beaten egg white into fruit purée before gently folding in remaining egg white. Spoon preparation into moulds, flattening the top gently with a knife. Place on a baking sheet and bake in oven for 12 to 15 mins.

Remove from oven, dust a little icing sugar on top, and serve immediately.

Raspberries with a pear and apple sauce

This dessert is very popular at our place and is best prepared in autumn at the beginning of the new apple and pear season when raspberries are still around. You can, of course, replace the raspberries with other fruits such as strawberries. It is special enough to serve to friends – stylish, yet simplicity itself to make.

SERVES 4

1 pear

1 apple

a few drops lemon juice

2 tbsp water

1 tsp sugar

2 tbsp low-fat natural yoghurt

1 tbsp low-fat milk

250 g (9 oz) raspberries

1 tsp bitter cocoa powder (optional)

Peel, quarter and core pear and apple. Halve apple pieces and place, along with pear, in a saucepan with lemon juice and water. Cook on medium heat until soft. Blend to a very fine purée with sugar. Allow to cool.

Whip yoghurt and milk for a few minutes to lighten it, then mix this into pear and apple purée.

Place raspberries in serving bowl and spoon pear and apple sauce on top. Shake the bowl.

Refrigerate until required, and dust with cocoa before serving.

Nectarine and rose-water salad

A delightful fruit salad for the family or to conclude the finest meal. The rose-water adds an exotic Middle Eastern flavour and is available from gourmet stores and some supermarkets and chemists.

SERVES 4

juice of 2 oranges

juice of ½ lemon

2 tsp rose-water

1 tbsp sugar

4 nectarines

2 William pears

2 tbsp chopped raw almonds

Combine orange juice, lemon juice, rose-water and sugar in a bowl.

Wash and halve nectarines. Slice them into segments and add to juice.

Wash, quarter and core pears, slice them, and add to bowl. Stir gently then refrigerate.

Remove from refrigerator about 30 mins before serving to allow fruit to return to room temperature. Sprinkle with almonds just before serving.

Nutty cherry and apple strudel

The first strudel was a variation on the Turkish baklava and was made by a Hungarian in Austria. It is a greatly loved, truly international dish. My version uses filo pastry. The secret of a good strudel is to ensure that the filling has as little moisture as possible.

SERVES 6

2 apples

2 tbsp castor sugar

1 tbsp sultanas

¼ tsp cinnamon

grated rind of ½ lemon

3 tbsp fresh breadcrumbs

1 tbsp chopped raw almonds

1 tbsp chopped walnuts

a 425 g (15 oz) can black pitted cherries, drained at least 1 hr in advance

4 sheets of wholemeal filo pastry

1–2 tbsp melted polyunsaturated margarine or butter

a little icing sugar from a shaker

Preheat oven to 200°C/400°F.

Peel, quarter, core and dice apples. Mix with sugar, sultanas, cinnamon, lemon rind, breadcrumbs, almonds, walnuts and cherries.

Spread a clean teatowel on your work bench. Place a sheet of filo pastry on towel and lightly brush it with melted margarine. Place a second sheet of pastry on top and brush again with a little melted margarine. Repeat procedure until you have no pastry left.

Spoon fruit mixture into the centre of the pastry and spread it out leaving an outside margin of about 5 cm (2 in) all round. Lift one of the longer sides of the cloth and roll pastry up completely.

Carefully place on a baking sheet and tuck the sides of the pastry underneath to seal the strudel well. Brush top with remaining margarine and make a few shallow cuts on top of pastry to allow any excess moisture to escape.

Bake in preheated oven for about 35 mins until pastry is crisp and golden brown. If pastry browns too much, lower temperature towards end of cooking. Transfer to cake rack, dust with icing sugar and serve hot or cold.

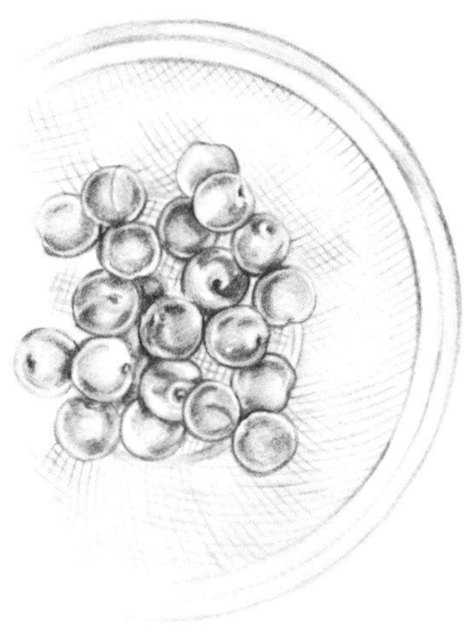

Kids Cooking

In the first years of life our taste preferences are modelled and greatly influenced by those who nourish us. Young children are naturally cautious about foods they have never tried, as they have no record of the flavour and texture of such foods. Since young children have a more sensitive flavour threshold (the point at which a stimulus is just strong enough to be perceived or to produce a response) than adults, the flavour of a new food can be overwhelming for them. It can take from several to many tastings for children to appreciate a new food and parents need not be overconcerned by repeated rejections. It is preferable to introduce food that is plainly cooked and without much seasoning, as this gives children the chance of registering the real flavour of the food and of learning to love natural flavours. The same type of food can be introduced in varied ways. For example, carrots can be served raw (whole, in sticks, grated, etc.) or cooked (whole, sliced, diced, puréed, etc.). Taste sensations often depend on texture, so a child may prefer a raw carrot to a cooked one.

We all have different tastes but it is important to remember that taste can be cultivated as we grow. The aim is for children to be introduced to a nutritionally balanced and wide variety of foods. However, children have the handicap of not knowing the words to describe their feelings, so they may say that such and such a food is 'yummy' or 'yukky' or they may simply say, 'I like it' or 'I don't like it', and they are usually unable to give reasons, making it difficult for parents to understand why they reject some foods.

Whether at home or at school, parents and teachers need to help children put their sensations into appropriate words. It is good to make children aware of the four classic tastes of sweetness, saltiness, acidity and bitterness. At the family table adults can point out when a taste is dominant or missing; for example, they can say, 'These strawberries are very sweet' or 'This orange is a little bitter' or 'This fruit juice is too acidic'. Children also need to be encouraged to discuss the shape, colour and texture of food as well as the sensations produced by the smell of food. All this knowledge helps them to become independent and gets them off to a good start in understanding what good food is about.

Children benefit greatly from shopping with adults, and for parents the assistance of children is helpful (they can also carry bags). Choosing good food is more easily learnt by example and parents can teach children as young as five or six years of age how to select good fruits and vegetables. Choosing meat and fish calls for a little more experience and discussion, but adults can point out the qualities or faults of a product by saying such things as 'Look how firm and shiny this fish is' or 'This fillet is still frozen; it is rock hard' or 'Those lamb chops have been well trimmed' or 'There is bone dust on those lamb chops', and so on. I believe this type of education gives future cooks great confidence. And once home from shopping, parents can show children where the various foods are stored.

Apart from cooking an occasional dish on their own, it is good for children to become familiar with the general skills of cooking, such as using equipment, lighting the oven, controlling the heat of the grill, operating the microwave, pouring hot milk from a saucepan into a cup, and so on. Children love to be useful in the kitchen and there are many little tasks they can do, such as peeling or cutting vegetables, filling a pot with water, adding pasta to boiling water and taking the scraps to the compost bin. When children do a particular task for the first time, say shelling peas, they need encouragement, and parents need to be patient. My eleven-year-old son can peel vegetables twice as fast now as he could a year ago. Parents' expectations should be consistent with the ability and maturity of the child. My children seem to enjoy the tasks we do together, as they can observe and practise at the same time. I am very grateful to my parents for the cooking skills they taught me in my childhood, for they have been the source of many great joys in the kitchen.

The following recipes have been specifically written for children six years old or above, and many children of even this age would need close parental supervision. It is potentially dangerous for young children to use sharp knives or gas and electrical appliances, or to handle hot liquids. *PGR* means 'parental guidance recommended', but you will find many recipes in the other chapters of this book that children can prepare or to which children can contribute, as most of the recipes are fast and easy.

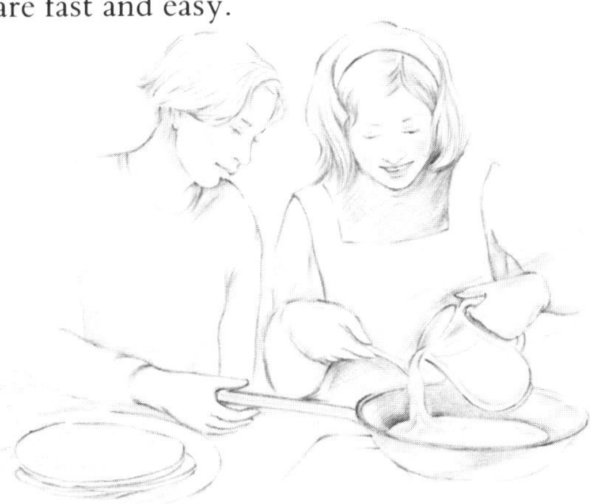

Hot chocolate   PGR*

This simple preparation that my children and I enjoy occasionally is a good way to learn to pour liquid from a saucepan. For this recipe you need a small saucepan, a cup and a teaspoon.

SERVES 1

1 cup low-fat milk

1 tsp cocoa

Remove milk from refrigerator and measure what you need into your cup. Pour milk into a small saucepan. Carefully place saucepan on stove and, with the aid of an adult, turn on heat under pan.

Measure cocoa into your cup. Close cocoa packet or tin well and put it back in the cupboard.

When milk starts to bubble at the edges and to form a skin on top, turn off heat. If the handle of the pan is hot and not heatproof, use an oven mitt to lift the pan. Carefully pour milk into your cup containing cocoa. Place the empty saucepan in the sink and add a little cold water to help with the washing up later.

Stir your hot chocolate and enjoy it.

Using a sponge, wipe any spilt milk or cocoa from the bench or table and wash any dirty dishes.

Peanut butter and grated carrot sandwich

When I give cooking classes to children, they seem to enjoy making and eating this sandwich more than any other. Try it and make one for your parents, too. They will be impressed with your skills. To prepare the sandwich you need a peeler, a grater, a chopping board and a knife to spread the peanut butter.

MAKES 2 SANDWICHES

1 medium carrot

4 slices wholegrain bread

about 2 tbsp peanut butter

Peel carrot. Grate carrot on the chopping board and place it on a small plate.

Place bread slices on board and spread two slices with peanut butter. Spread grated carrot on the other two slices and top these two with the first two slices, placing the peanut butter side down. Press lightly on the bread using the flat of your hand and cut each sandwich in half. Arrange sandwiches on plates and serve.

Wash the dishes and board and wipe the bench after enjoying your creation.

**Parental guidance recommended*

Pita bread, ham and pineapple pizza   PGR

Ham and pineapple pizza is a favourite with kids. Feel free to prepare a topping of your choice and remember that the ingredients you use must not be too moist or the pizza base will become soggy during the cooking. To prepare this dish you need a flat oven tray, serrated knife, can opener, chopping board, grater, two plates and an egg lifter. Ask an adult to help with the cooking of the pizza.

SERVES 1

1 small slice pita bread

1 slice pineapple, fresh or canned

1 tbsp grated low-fat mozzarella cheese

1 thin slice ham

1 small tomato

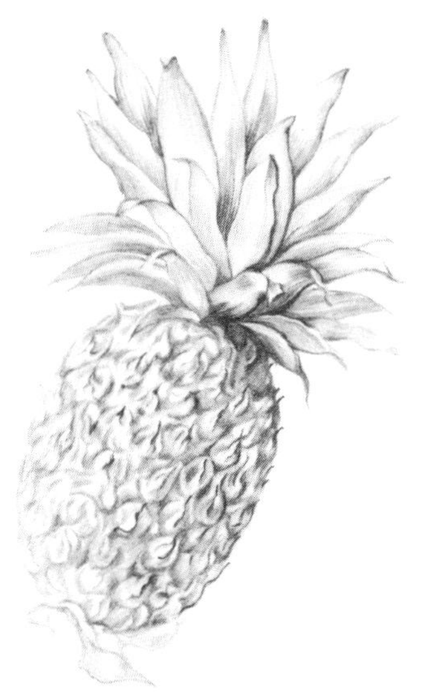

Preheat oven to 220°C/450°F.

Place pita bread on oven tray.

Open can of pineapple, remove one slice and put on a plate.

Grate cheese onto a plate.

Roll up slice of ham and cut thinly into pieces.

Cut pineapple slice first in half, then into quarters, then cut each quarter into three pieces. Place pineapple pieces on plate.

Wash tomato and cut into 1 cm (⅓ in) thick slices. Arrange tomato slices on pita bread without overlapping. You may not need them all. Then sprinkle with about half the grated cheese. Scatter pieces of ham on top and then arrange pineapple pieces on top of ham. Lastly, add remaining grated cheese.

With the help of an adult and using an oven mitt, place pizza in preheated oven and cook for about 10 mins or until cheese is well melted.

Again with the aid of an adult and using an oven mitt, remove pizza tray from oven. Place in a safe place, such as on top of the stove. Remember, it is hot and others could burn themselves. Turn oven off.

Using an egg lifter, lift pizza onto a plate and enjoy it!

Remember to wash the dishes after your meal.

Pancakes   PGR

When I was a child we made pancakes as a treat for special occasions. It is best to mix a pancake batter at least 30 mins before cooking the pancakes. They can be served with some sliced fruit wrapped inside and the top can be dusted with icing sugar. I'm sure your parents will enjoy giving you a hand with the cooking, if necessary. To prepare this dish, you need a medium mixing bowl, a whisk, a jug, a frying pan or pancake pan, and a wide spatula or egg lifter.

MAKES ABOUT 6 PANCAKES

½ cup plain white flour

½ cup plain wholemeal flour

1 egg

1½ cups low-fat milk

a small pinch of salt

1 tsp peanut oil

1 tsp polyunsaturated margarine or butter

Place both types of flour in bowl and make a hollow in the centre. Into the hollow pour egg, half of the milk and the salt. Using a whisk, first mix egg and milk together then gradually incorporate flour, slowly adding the rest of the milk to form a smooth mixture. Refrigerate for at least 30 mins before using.

Pour pancake batter into a jug that pours well.

You might like to ask an adult to help you for this part and for the following steps. Heat oil and margarine in frying pan. Pour hot oil and melted margarine into pancake batter and mix well.

Return pan to heat. Pour a little batter into pan to thinly cover the base of the pan. Twirl pan smoothly to form a thin, even pancake. When the top half of the pancake starts to dry a bit, turn pancake over using a wide spatula. Then cook the second side for about 1 min and remove pancake. Start cooking another immediately without adding any more margarine or oil to pan. After making the last pancake, turn off heat.

Enjoy your pancakes and remember to wash the dishes and wipe the bench and stove.

Bananatana salad

To prepare this dessert or snack, you need a chopping board, a hand juicer, a medium mixing bowl, a small serrated knife and a large spoon. It is easier to work on the kitchen table rather than a bench, which is often too high and not comfortable for children.

SERVES 2

1 orange

1 tbsp sultanas

2 small bananas

Hold orange with one hand on chopping board and cut it in half. Squeeze orange juice with a hand juicer and pour juice into bowl. Add sultanas to juice.

Peel bananas on chopping board. Cut bananas into small slices and add to bowl. Using a large spoon, gently stir banana with juice. This stops the banana from darkening in colour.

The dish is now ready. If not using within 15 mins, cover bowl and refrigerate.

Wash chopping board, hand juicer, knife and spoon and put fruit skins into compost or rubbish bin. Don't forget to wipe the bench.

Index